2 10 27.

RC
627
.S7
A43
1979

American Jewish Joint Distribution
   Committee.
   Hunger disease : studies / by the
Jewish physicians in the Warsaw ghetto
; edited by Myron Winick ; translated
from the Polish by Martha Osnos. -- New
York : Wiley, c1979.
   xiv, 261 p. : ill. ; 24 cm. --
(Current concepts in nutrition ; v. 7)

Hunger Disease

CURRENT CONCEPTS IN NUTRITION

Myron Winick, Editor

Institute of Human Nutrition
Columbia University College of Physicians and Surgeons

HUNGER DISEASE

STUDIES BY THE JEWISH PHYSICIANS IN THE WARSAW GHETTO

Edited by

Myron Winick, M.D.
R. R. Williams Professor of Nutrition
Professor of Pediatrics
Director of the Institute of Human Nutrition
Columbia University College of Physicians and Surgeons

Translated from the Polish by
Martha Osnos, Research Associate
Columbia University College of Physicians and Surgeons

A WILEY-INTERSCIENCE PUBLICATION

JOHN WILEY & SONS, New York · Chichester · Brisbane · Toronto

The original Polish manuscript printed by the
American Joint Distribution Committee,
Warsaw, 1946

Library of Congress Cataloging in Publication Data:

American Jewish Joint Distribution Committee.
    Hunger disease.

    (Current concepts in nutrition; v. 7)
    Translation of Choroba glodowa.
    "A Wiley-Interscience publication."
    Includes index.
    1. Deficiency diseases.   2. Malnutrition.   3.   Jews
in Warsaw—Persecutions.   4.   Holocaust, Jewish (1939–
1945)—Poland—Warsaw.   5.   Starvation.   6.   Hunger.
I. Winick, Myron,   II.   Title.   III.   Series.

RC623.5.A43   1979   616.3'9   78–26397
ISBN 0–471–05003–2

EDITORIAL COMMITTEE

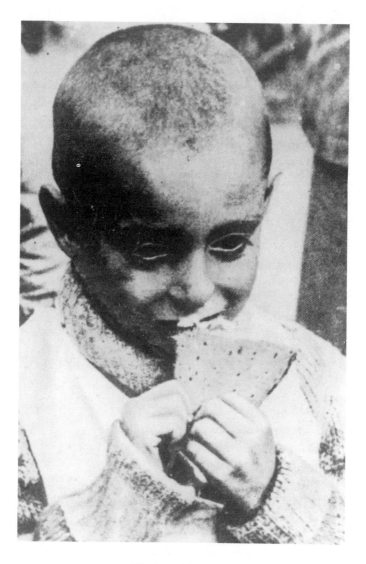

The face of hunger.

PREFACE

The book you are about to read is one that is, and that we can only hope will remain, unique in the annals of medicine. It is the report of a scientific study by physicians condemned to die of the same disease they were studying—hunger and subsequent starvation. The time was 1940, the place the Jewish ghetto in Warsaw, Poland. The Nazis had sealed several hundred thousand people off from the outside world, determined to starve them to death. Amid the destruction, starvation, and rampant infectious disease a group of physicians decided to undertake a careful medical investigation of the clinical, metabolic, and pathologic consequences of hunger and starvation. To undertake such a study in a fully equipped hospital using a well trained staff would have been difficult enough; to undertake the study in a hospital within the ghetto walls which was poorly equipped and staffed by personnel who themselves were starving was remarkable. The details of the study had to be worked out in secret meetings, the essential equipment had to be smuggled into the ghetto, personnel had to be trained, and the entire operation had to be kept secret from Nazi conquerors who wanted none of this exposed to the outside world. Even the final manuscript had to be smuggled out to the Aryan side. It was entrusted to Professor Orlowski, Director of the Department of Medicine at Warsaw University, who buried it until it could be safely uncovered.

The major figure in the organization of these studies was Dr. Israel Milejkowski, the Jewish physician responsible for public health in the ghetto. He felt that it was necessary for the world to know the extent and the crippling consequences of the starvation being imposed. He proposed that the effects be documented by the best medical minds in the ghetto, the same physicians who were directing the various services in the hospitals where attempts were being made to rehabilitate these patients. In an initial meeting he gathered together Dr. Emil Apfelbaum, the Chief of Cardiology at the Czyste Hospital and a well known authority on diseases of the circulation; Dr. Julian Fliederbaum, a graduate of the University of Petrograd, an internist from Vilna, who had come to Warsaw as a refugee, and who was now director of the hospital on Stawki Street; Dr. Anna Braude-Heller, perhaps the most renowned Jewish pediatrician in Poland, the moving spirit in the development of the Medem Sanitarium, and later the medical director of the Bauman-Berson Children's Hospital; Dr. Mieczyslaw Kocen, a native of Lodz, and a specialist in blood diseases; and Dr. Joseph Stein, a renowned pathologist, a holder of both a PhD and a medical degree, who in spite of his conversion to Catholicism many years before was forced into the ghetto. He was now Director of the Czyste Hospital, the largest and best known Jewish hospital in Poland. Although only these six physicians attended the initial organizing meeting, there were ultimately 28 physicians who played a major role in the implementation of the study. The fates of these physician-scientists were uniformly tragic. Milejkowski and Fliederbaum committed suicide; Kocen and Stein were exterminated in Treblinka. Braude-Heller was killed in a bunker during the uprising while resisting to the end. Apfelbaum survived long enough to recover the manuscript and prepare it for publication, only to die of a heart attack on a Warsaw street in 1946 at the age of 56. The manuscript, however, survived and was published simultaneously in limited Polish and French editions in 1946 by the American Joint Distribution Committee. It was known and cited by some researchers in the late 1940s and early 1950s. However, because of limited availability, it somehow was lost from the general medical literature. Dr. William Schmidt, then the director of the AJDC's health department, and Dr. Aleksander Gonik, its present director, tried to have the report translated and given wider dissemination all through these years. In fact, it was Dr. Schmidt who had brought a copy out to the United States after its printing in Warsaw. In 1966 Dr. Leonard Tushnet, a general practitioner in New Jersey, published a summary of the findings and an account of the participating physicians in a monograph entitled *The Uses of Adversity—Studies of Starvation in the Warsaw Ghetto*. The manuscript itself surfaced again about two years ago, when its existence was mentioned in an article in the *New England Journal of Medicine*. I first heard about it from a physician at Columbia Presbyterian Medical Center whose wife had seen a copy on a visit to Poland. She contacted Morris Laub, the executive chairman of the

YIVO Institute for Jewish Research, who found a copy in the archives and asked me if I thought it was worth translating into English. After consultation with a colleague who reads Polish, it was decided to go ahead. Mrs. Martha Osnos, a research associate at the Institute of Human Nutrition of Columbia University College of Physicians and Surgeons, whose father was one of the best known and most widely respected Jewish physicians in Warsaw, and who knew some of these doctors personally, undertook the translation. On May 24, 1978, a major symposium was held at the College of Physicians and Surgeons in New York honoring the physicians of the Warsaw ghetto and reporting the most important findings of the study.

The studies that are reported are fragmented and incomplete—fragmented because several manuscripts were either never written owing to the death of the principal investigator or lost beneath the rubble of the destroyed ghetto following the uprising which led to the final annihilation of the Jews of Warsaw; incomplete because the Nazis, not satisfied with slow starvation as an efficient method of liquidation of the Jewish population of Warsaw, began a policy of massive deportation in July 1942, which effectively ended the investigations. The hospitals were closed and the personnel, including many of the physicians conducting the studies, were deported to concentration camps, where most were relieved of their own starvation disease in the gas chambers. And yet, fragmented and incomplete as they are, these studies represent a true milestone in medical research, for they demonstrate what the determination of a handful of dedicated physicians could accomplish using their training and experience, their ingenuity, and the resources they could muster.

Because of the unique population that was available for study, observations could be made which had never been made before and some of which have never been made since. The design of the studies was of necessity cross sectional; the patients were carefully selected to represent pure hunger disease without complicating infections such as typhus or tuberculosis, which were both rampant in the population. The actual studies undertaken were based on three considerations: the importance of the information to be obtained, the areas of expertise of available investigators, and the possibility of carrying out the studies properly under existing conditions. The studies therefore represent a curious mixture. The clinical observations in both children and adults constitute probably the best clinical description of the effects of severe semistarvation published in the medical literature to that date and perhaps even to the present. The precise description of the skin changes, the nature and pathogenesis of the edema, the appearance of effusions in various body cavities, the changes in temperature, blood pressure, and pulse rate are noted with great care. The description of how the patients lie in bed, how they move, their reaction to outside stimuli can be considered almost classic. Some of these clinical observations, as will be pointed out in the comments dealing with the individual chapters, were original at the time they were made. A few remain unique today.

The metabolic studies were extremely focused. Those on carbohydrate metabolism, to my knowledge, are the most extensive ever carried out on that subject. The studies on acid base balance were also quite extensive and will certainly add new knowledge to the medical literature. Other studies, such as those on nitrogen and mineral metabolism, while incomplete, were meticulously carried out and some of the findings, when added to those of later studies, help fill gaps in our knowledge.

The investigations into the circulatory changes are again extremely sophisticated and used certain techniques actually devised by the principal investigator. Measurements were made of blood volume, arterial and venous pressure, and general and capillary circulation times. In addition electrocardiographic studies and studies of the circulatory response to certain drugs were carefully carried out. The investigators also studied the distribution of water and electrolytes between the intracellular, extracellular, and vascular spaces. Finally, an interpretation of the circulatory changes in hunger disease is put forth. This interpretation, for the most part, still stands today.

The studies on blood and bone marrow are revealing, not so much from the standpoint of the actual research findings but more from the standpoint of the results of various therapeutic trials. The investigators were above all physicians, dedicated to the art of healing. Nowhere in this entire manuscript is this more evident than in the chapter on blood. The doctors were trying desperately to cure the anemia they were confronting. They employed every mode of therapy available to them—iron, liver, the combination of both, as well as small transfusions of blood. None of them worked. In fact, in some cases the situation became worse and the patients' condition deteriorated. But they tried, and this was what their training and their expertise demanded.

The report on the eye findings is unique, probably because of the availability of a team of well trained ophthalmologists who realized the importance of making these observations and measurements on patients suffering from hunger disease. A part of the manuscript that dealt with detailed studies of fields of vision was lost. This is a great loss to medical science, since it is unlikely that such studies will ever be repeated. The remainder of the manuscript describes in detail a number of clinical and pathophysiological observations on the eye, which to my knowledge are completely new to the medical literature.

The final chapter depicts the grim reality of what these physician-scientists were facing, through autopsy reports and reports of macroscopic and microscopic examination of tissues. The statistics garnered from these studies document, as had never been documented before, the gross organ changes in semistarvation. The detailed descriptions are the work of an obviously well trained and careful pathologist. The histologic studies had just begun when the deportations and the destruction of the hospital took place. The few reports begin to develop a pattern but the details could not be worked out.

The book in its entirety is important for reasons beyond science and medicine, for through the kind of work they did we can learn about at least a part of the character of these physicians. They were all well trained, all specialists in their fields. They had read the literature available. Some, such as Drs. Fliederbaum and Apfelbaum, were trained scientists, and their scientific background and ingenuity come through clearly. Another, Dr. Milejkowski, was an organizer and coordinator, and undoubtedly kept the team going through periods of great adversity. The others were clinicians primarily, but in the old sense—able to observe critically and to inquire about what they observed. What they accomplished together was truly remarkable. It is tempting to speculate on the character of these men and women outside their credentials as physicians. What made them obsessively carry out these studies, carefully note their findings, and prepare and preserve their manuscript? Was it the challenge? Was it a way to keep their sanity? Was it a need to leave something to posterity? Perhaps someday this aspect of the drama will be revealed.

The real heroes of this book, however, are the Jews of Warsaw. For in their despair and from their suffering they have left the world a legacy. From history's bleakest period of man's inhumanity to man come not only the moral lessons which will be with us for ages but a scientific and medical message which may contribute to the ultimate betterment of mankind. With the publication of this book, I hope, their last wish has been accomplished—*Non omnis moriar*—I shall not wholly die!

MYRON WINICK, M.D.

New York
March 1979

CONTENTS

Introduction

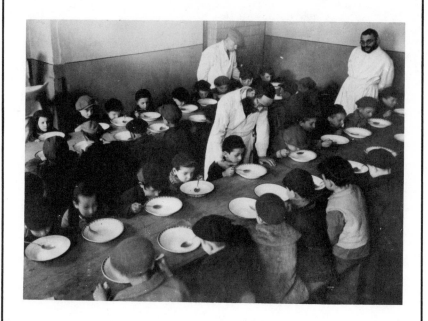

*Soup kitchen for feeding children. From the archives of the
YIVO Institute for Jewish Research, reproduced by permission.*

The torture of words . . . I have never felt it as strongly as now when I have to write an introduction to this work. This is an unbelievable moment since the work was originated and pursued under unbelievable conditions. I hold my pen in my hand and death stares into my room. It looks through the black windows of sad empty houses on deserted streets littered with vandalized and burglarized possessions. It is difficult under such conditions to collect one's wits and even more difficult to express one's feelings. My tongue is too pallid to present the magnitude of the defeat. I am looking for suitable words—it is torture.

This work was never finished. It was interrupted on July 22, 1942. This was a crucial day in the history of the Warsaw ghetto—the day when the deportations, the mass murder, began. Yes, deportations, mass murder, synonymous words in the history of the ghetto. The monstrosity of it will be fully understood only in the future.

Let us be silent—as silent as the empty houses in the empty streets of our ghetto. In this prevailing silence lies the power and the depth of our pain and the moans that one day will shake the world's conscience.

The history of the Warsaw ghetto can be divided into two periods—before July 22, 1942 and the period following. The first period was characterized by general hunger, the second period by massive death. It is not surprising, therefore, that when the second period started, the work on hunger stopped. The hospitals and laboratories were destroyed and, most important, the human element, our workers and the subjects of our work, were gone. Work was stopped but not liquidated. When the first horrible shock of the deportations was over, the accumulated scientific material was studied again and organized. This is the work being published now. It is an "unfinished symphony" full of meaning, written by Jewish doctors in 1942. One detail should not be omitted: the work on the manuscript is being carried out in one of the undestroyed rooms of the cemetery buildings. This is the symbol of our living and working environment.

The work on hunger started in February 1942. Hunger was the most important factor of everyday life within the walls of the Warsaw ghetto. Its symptoms consisted of crowds of beggars and corpses often lying on the streets covered with newspapers. Mortality data on hunger and its two companions, tuberculosis and typhus, were collected from orphanages and refugee centers and from specific hospital material.

A group of medical colleagues, themselves living constantly with the hunger problem, decided that the reality of their everyday grim life should become the subject of our scientific work. Disregarding the terrible conditions, which were completely unsuitable to the work in progress, all of these doctors labored with utmost devotion and fervor. The hospitals were located in temporary buildings not suitable for the purpose, and lack of apparatus, reagents, and other equipment made the research even more difficult. Many of our physician colleagues themselves suffered from hunger. In spite of this, nobody interrupted the work and quietly, modestly, without any advertising the work was done. The material collected during five months would have required at least a year under normal conditions. It was as if we knew subconsciously that the work could be interrupted at any minute.

The tops of the walls of the Warsaw ghetto were covered with broken glass. Their purpose was singular: mass extermination by mass starvation. That was the reason for this odious brick and glass structure. But the creator of this monstrosity was somehow frustrated; a new unpredicted power arose in Warsaw: smuggling. Smuggling, a rather shameful occupation, was our salvation. Night and day the smugglers fought the diabolic forces that built the walls. Smuggling food from the Aryan part of Warsaw curtailed the prevalence of hunger, its spread, its tempo, and its irreversibility. No changes in the structure of the walls—no bricks, no maiming broken glass—could prevent some supplies from trickling into the ghetto. Therefore the enemy had to find another more efficient means of extermination.

After 18 months of struggle our conqueror, seeking our possessions, our blood, and our lives, discovered a better way and hunger was replaced by deportation.

Deportation became the curse of the ghetto. Where to? How? People were chased from the streets, from apartments, from basements and attics. They were chased with guns and with whips into the unknown. Packed into cattletrains, children separated from parents and wives from husbands, masses of people without water or bread. People driven in inhuman chaos, disorganized, the old, the young, the healthy, and the mortally sick together; a trip without return. This system of extermination was much more efficient than hunger; we have the data to prove it.

The closing of the ghetto walls resulted in 43,000 deaths; in two months deportation resulted in 250,000 deaths. Therefore I emphasize once more the role of the unknown smuggler, who with his own blood and sweat made our scientific work in the ghetto possible.

I must mention here two men who helped us to start and to continue our research, the head of the Jewish council, Adam Czerniakow, and the head of the economic council, Abraham Gepner.

A last few words to honor you, the Jewish doctors. What can I tell you, my beloved colleagues and companions in misery. You are a part of all of us. Slavery, hunger, deportation, those death figures in our ghetto were also your legacy. And you by your work could give the henchman the answer "Non omnis moriar," "I shall not wholly die."

DR. ISRAEL MILEJKOWSKI

Head, Department of Public Health
Jewish Council in Warsaw
Warsaw, October 1942

Participating
Physicians

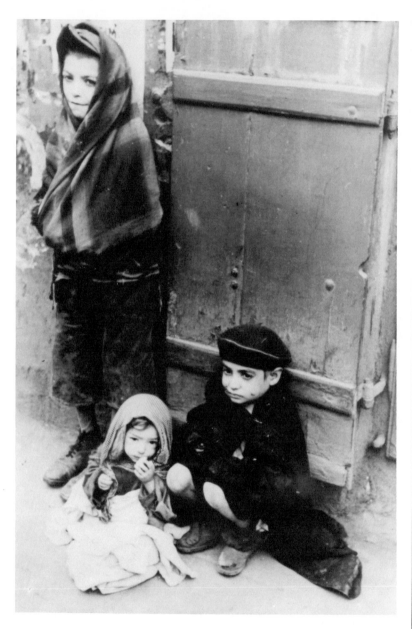

A hungry family on a ghetto street. From the archives of the YIVO Institute for Jewish Research, reproduced by permission.

Dr. Roza Amzel—*died 1943.*
Dr. Emil Apfelbaum—*died 1946.*
Dr. Zdzislaw Askanas—*survived.*
Dr. Owsiej Bielenki—*died 1943.*
Dr. Leon Blacher—*died 1942.*
Dr. Anna Braude-Heller—*died 1943.*
Dr. Chaim Einhorn—*survived.*
Dr. Regina Elbinger—*died 1943.*
Dr. Szymon Fajgenblat—*died 1944.*
Dr. Henryk Fenigstein—*survived.*
Fajga Ferszt—*died 1942.*
Dr. Julian Fliederbaum—*died 1943.*
Dr. Teodosie Goliborska—*survived.*
Dr. Ari Heller—*survived.*
Jerzy Herzekruk—*died 1943.*
Dr. Mieczyslaw Kocen—*died 1943.*
Dr. Israel Milejkowski—*died 1943.*
Dr. Ryszard Pakszwer—*died 1943.*
Dr. Moryc Plonskier—*died 1942.*
Dr. Boleslaw Raszkes—*died 1942.*
Dr. Israel Rotbalsam—*survived.*
Dr. Joseph Stein—*died 1943.*
Suzanne Szejnfinkel—*unknown.*
Dr. Mieczyslaw Szejnman—*died 1943.*
Dr. Michal Szejnman—*died 1492.*
Dr. Ichaskil Wohl—*died 1943.*
Jeanne Zarchi—*died 1942.*
Dr. Kazimierz Zweibaum—*survived.*

ONE   Clinical Aspects of Hunger Disease in Adults

Dr. Julian Fliederbaum

with the collaboration of

Dr. Ari Heller

Dr. Kazimierz Zweibaum

Jeanne Zarchi

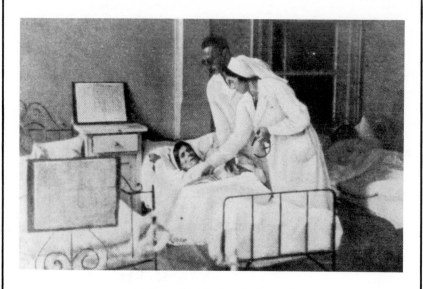

Adult ward in the Jewish Hospital.

Hunger is as old as the history of mankind. We know of hunger in China, in Russia, during the Civil War, and in Germany during World War I. Still, the clinical aspects and the biochemistry of continuous hunger as well as the pathogenesis of the symptoms are not very well described. Because of the inappropriate conditions for conducting scientific work, the clinical aspects of hunger edema were not carefully investigated during the 1914-18 war. We will try to extend what studies there have been using the latest scientific methods.

Our studies were carried out from February to July 1942 in the departments of medicine and pediatrics of the Jewish Hospital Czyste in Warsaw, Poland. The studies include 70 adult clinic patients, about 40 children, and some 30 people seen as private patients. The adults had been kept on a very low calorie diet, with small amounts of protein and fat, for several months, some even for years. According to the data obtained from the department of supply in the Warsaw ghetto, the 800 calorie diet contained 3 g of fat and 20 to 30 g of vegetable protein. It consisted of dark bread, rye flour, kasha, potatoes, traces of butter, lard, oil, sugar, and a plateful of soup. It contained mostly carbohydrates and was grossly deficient in vitamins.

We included in our studies patients who had no obvious complications such as tuberculosis, hunger diarrhea, abscesses, and avitaminosis. We could confirm our diagnoses very often by comparing them later with the autopsy reports.

These so-called clean cases were the background on which the abovementioned complications occurred. We have attempted to clarify the following clinical questions:

1. Why do some diseases occur very rarely and others quite commonly during hunger disease?
2. Why do some diseases follow an atypical course during war and hunger?
3. How can spontaneous recoveries in certain patients with hunger disease be explained?

4. What is the etiology of the edema, marasmus, tetany, and premature aging?
5. What is the mechanism of death?

The studies that follow are an attempt to clarify the clinical aspects and biochemical and physiological findings in these five areas.

CASE HISTORIES AND INTERVIEWS

Constant thirst and persistent increase in urinary output (4 to 5 liters) with fixed specific gravity of the urine are the first signs of even a short period of hunger or of a drastic change in the diet as occurred during the war. Generally, the urge to urinate does not prevent sleep. However, during hunger disease the patients have to get up during the night. Other early complaints include dryness in the mouth, rapid weight loss, and a constant craving for food.

With prolonged hunger, these symptoms diminish. The patients now experience general weakness and the inability to sustain even the smallest physical effort, and are unwilling to work. They remain in bed all day, covered because they always feel cold, most acutely in the nose and the extremities. They become apathetic and depressed, and lack initiative. They do not remember their hunger, but when shown bread, meat, or sweets they become very aggressive, grab the food, and devour it at once, even though they may be beaten for it and have no strength to run away. Toward the end of hunger disease the only complaint is complete exhaustion.

Even in apparently healthy individuals the symptoms may differ. Cardiovascular symptoms include easy tiring while climbing stairs, but no cardiac anxiety or dyspnea. Respiratory symptoms, such as the tendency to catch cold and to cough, with several forms of expectorate, are quite common. Gastrointestinal complaints include the appearance of very bulky stools and a tendency to mucous and bloody discharge from the colon, which is often the cause of death. Very often edema appears, and for this reason hunger disease has also been called edema disease. Edema usually appears first on the face, followed by swelling of the feet and legs, especially in individuals who walk or stand a great deal. In the early stages of hunger disease edema disappears during bed rest. In the late stages edema affects the whole body.

Initially the large urinary output and constant thirst are dominant but these symptoms disappear in the later stages of hunger. There are complaints of aches and pains in the ribs, the sternum, the pelvis, and the lower extremities, and of nervousness and anxiety, but few psychic abnormalities. Women miss their menstrual periods and are sterile. Men are impotent and the few children who are born die within a few weeks.

By simply observing these patients one can see their characteristic posture, where flexors dominate over extensors, just like a fetus in the womb. This is sometimes due to existing contractures. The patients are always sleepy, always cold. Regardless of season they lie motionless, covered with blankets and pillows.

The body structure of people who were still growing during the three years of war and hunger is very delicate and asthenic, almost like filigree. Their height is much below normal, their bones are narrow, and their chests are often flat. They show double *vertebra prominens,* moveable tenth rib, and dichotomy of the spinous processes of the lumbar vertebra.

Weights, which were recorded very carefully, ranged from 30 to 40 kg, which is 20 to 50% less than normal for the hospital population before the war. Considering that a hospital population usually is below normal weight, the values are even more striking. One woman, 30 years old, 152 cm tall, weighed 24 kg. There was almost complete atrophy of adipose tissue.

Three degrees of emaciation were observed:

1. Disappearance of surplus fat. This stage was reminiscent of the time before the war when people went to Marienbad, Karlsbad, or Vichy for a reducing cure and came back looking younger and feeling better.

2. A stage in which the patients looked old and withered, as was the case with most of our patients.
3. Hunger cachexia in the terminal stage.

We shall now describe specific changes in the organs affected by hunger disease. Dr. B. Raszkes' manuscript on the skin unfortunately was lost, and hence we shall summarize his chief observations. The color of the skin is characteristically pale or cyanotic. The skin is covered with dirty brown pigment, either in small clusters or diffusely distributed, similar to pigmentation of suprarenal origin but with a different localization. Rarely is the pigment localized in places exposed to sunshine, or in the usual physiological locations such as abdomen's ligament, Hunter's line, nipples, around the armpits and the genital areas, the face, the palms, and the soles. On the contrary, it concentrates around the neck, the rump, on the sides of the torso, except for the armpits, and on the back of the arms and the thighs. It is a real *cutis vagabondarum*. In those patients with hunger disease who were seen in private practice, the skin is unusually pale, almost whitish. The hospital population is usually very poor and also very dirty as a result of the terrible sanitary conditions in the ghetto. The skin is infested with parasites such as lice, scabies, and crusted ringworm, and dermatoses, furunculoses, subdermal abscesses, and diffuse phlegmones are very common. Lice and dermatoses cause itching and the scratched skin is excoriated and traumatized.

We do not believe that the hyperpigmentation results from malnutrition but rather that the pigment localizes in traumatized areas of skin. In the third stage of hunger the face becomes cachexic and dirty brown. In some rare cases even the conjunctiva and the sides of the tongue have this dirty brown hue. The skin is chapped and dry. There is atrophy of sweat glands and no pilometric reflexes. The cuticle becomes parakeratotic or, less often, hyperkeratotic. When the skin is rubbed with a fingernail a large scar appears at once. Sometimes if a patient scratches his front in the morning, a long scaly and flaky scar remains until evening. This characteristic symptom appears also on the back, the frontal part of the breast, and the arms and thighs. The skin is very thin, atrophic, wrinkled, and devoid of elasticity and turgor. It looks like cigarette paper or old parchment.

When adipose tissue starts to disappear and skinfolds become shallower, the faces of hungry people look younger, but in the second and even more in the third stage, men and especially women look very old. This is the result of complete cachexia, pigmentation, thinning, wrinkling and dryness, and the parchment look of the skin.

Temperature varies in different parts of the body. As a rule the extremities are very cold. Sweat glands are atrophied, and palms and fingertips are never moist. This is the first degree of dryness. The second degree of dryness is characterized by flaky parakeratosis. In the third degree a skinfold once formed with fingers does not go back; it just remains folded. Our patients showed mainly the first and second degrees of dryness.

The sebaceous glands are hardly active. There is no seborrhea; there are no enlarged pores and no blackheads.

Hair growth is abnormal. If puberty occurs during the hunger period the hair grows very luxuriantly on the head and in the genital regions. Mustache and whiskers appear, as do long eyelashes, hairy supraciliar arches, and luxuriant fuzz all over the body. People 30 to 50 years old, on the contrary, lose their hair, even in the armpits and the genital regions. When the hair is cut short it looks like bristle; it is thick, stiff, and uneven. Fingernails are dull and have longitudinal or latitudinal stripes. They are clawlike and show a tendency to paronychiae.

Although the skin is dry, the underlying tissue is waterlogged. Pasty edema starts mostly in the face, around the eyelids, as in kidney disease, or in some people in the feet and ankles, as in heart disease. It subsides during bed rest. Some people develop edema in the scrotum and labia majorae. The extent and degree of edema are very variable. If the edema subsides after one day in bed in the hospital we call it first degree waterlogging. In patients who have atrophy of skinfolds in the face, the Aldrich-McClure water test often proved that water absorption from the skin is increased. The water blister that normally disappears in this test after 60 minutes, disappeared in these patients after 20 to 30 minutes. We called this stage second degree waterlogging. Third degree waterlogging is characterized by really severe edema with fluid in the pleural cavity, the peritoneal cavity, and sometimes in the pericardial cavity. Pressing the flesh with a finger results in a dimple lasting 1 to 5 minutes (2 minutes on the sole). The Aldrich-McClure blister disappears in 10 minutes. A puncture yields fluid from subcutaneous tissue. The edematous swellings change in locale depending on the patient's position in bed.

In addition to the abovementioned conditions in skin we noted widespread hypersensitivity toward sunrays in spring. Redness, swelling, local hyperthermia, and fever blisters appear even after one session in the sun. This is real *acrodermatitis actinica*. In early fall there are cases of frostbite of the fingers and toes and sometimes third degree frostbite of the forearms and feet.

The general body temperature is lower than normal; instead of 36.6° it is 35.2° to 35.3°. For example in typhus, usually characterized by high fever, among other symptoms, the temperature often remains low. Patients complain of feeling cold.

The lymph nodes are not generally enlarged, and if they are it usually is the result of tuberculosis. Tuberculosis is now very prevalent, unlike before the war, and has rapidly spread throughout the population. The cachexic patients usually die not from tuberculosis, which does not have time to invade the lungs, but from hunger disease.

Skeletal muscles are slack and atrophic, their activity diminished. All movements are slow. These are all symptoms of bradykinesis. Because of technical difficulties we could not measure the functional disabilities of the extremities in these patients but we observed their weakness, their slow movements at work, their clumsy attempts to grab a piece of bread from the doctor's hand, their running which always resulted in a fall. We examined urine for creatinine and creatine in 24 hour samples from 20 adults. It contained normal or slightly low levels of creatinine, but in 17 samples we discovered the presence of creatine.

In normal samples creatine appears after great muscular effort, or after muscular decomposition in endocrine disturbances such as hypoparathyroidism or castration.

These patients have a characteristic masklike appearance. Their faces are expressionless and pale. The conjunctivae are spotted with brown and the thin sclerae are blue. Ophthalmologic examinations did not detect Bitot spots, softening of the cornea, or night blindness. The pupils are narrow and round and often react sluggishly to light. We explain this finding as the result of flabbiness of the sphincter of the iris.

Premature changes in the lens similar to those seen in senile cataracts were observed. The normal intraocular pressure is 20 to 30 mm Hg. In hunger cachexia it can be as low as 12 mm Hg. Hearing and sense of equilibrium were normal.

Some patients have *angulus infectiosus oris*. The mucosa of the mouth cavity is normal. The tongue is mostly coated, and patients complain of a burning sensation. The base of the tongue is smooth, as a result of atrophy of papillae, and sometimes the tongue appears inflamed and blistered. The teeth are in bad condition. Dental caries are extremely prevalent and changes occur around the apex of the roots. People as young as 20 often cannot chew their food because of these changes.

The gums do not show the characteristics of vitamin C deficiency. The tonsils are usually atrophied. Tonsillitis, like scarlet fever, was rare during World War II, but according to the pediatricians, diphtheria is more frequent and often more virulent.

In the terminal stage of cachexia and marasmus the voice becomes hoarse, like *vox cholerica* or *carcinomatosa*. We could not ascertain whether this is due to organic causes, such as changes in the innervation of the larynx, or to functional changes secondary to dehydration. When starvation occurs in boys during puberty the voice does not undergo the usual changes.

The two lobes of the thyroid are more prominent than normally, owing to the thinness of the neck. In one case we observed enlarged parotid glands without signs of inflammation.

The chest in young adults is asthenic whereas it is normal or sometimes barrel shaped in elderly people.

We were especially careful in examining the lungs. Regardless of the shape of the chest, at percussion we found high pitched tympanic resonance all over the lungs and a lowering of the lung borders sometimes until the twelfth costal rib. The heart borders were overlapped by lung tissue, making it difficult to establish the real borders of the heart through dullness of percussion. There was normal mobility of the lower borders of the lung during deep inspiration and little mobility during shallow inspiration.

According to Neuman's principle, tympanic resonance in an asthenic chest is a sign of pulmonary tuberculosis. However, in the few cases where X-rays were available we could demonstrate radiolucency of the lungs, free costophrenic angles, lowering of the lower lung borders, and decreased pulmonary mobility in the absence of tubercular signs. This new syndrome of atony of the lungs, never before described in hunger disease, was characteristic and consistent in the lungs of our patients.

Tuberculosis of the caseous, ulcerative, cavitating, or fulminating variety has long been known to occur in conjunction with long term starvation. There was a great increase in tuberculosis during the war. We tried to determine why hunger disease is accompanied by active primary or secondary tuberculosis. We concluded that among the factors responsible are atony of the lungs, decreased muscle tonus, and impaired ventilation, mostly in the apex. We made the following observations in 20 carefully examined cases: lung capacity decreased by 1½ to 3 liters, rate of respiration decreased to 11 to 12 per minute, and volume of air intake also decreased. We observed, too, that poor blood circulation, impaired capillarization secondary to defects in the circulatory system, and decreased immunity contributed to the high incidence of active tuberculosis. Even during World War I it was known that blood with a low level of fat was deficient as a carrier of antibodies.

In the tuberculosis department we tried to determine the sensitivity of the host to tuberculin. We used the allergenic method of Dr. F. Groer as modified for adults by Dr. W. Hartwig in Prof. W. Orlowski's clinic. Twenty patients with pure hunger disease and 40 patients with pulmonary and pleural tuberculosis were injected intradermally with 0.1 cc of Koch old tuberculin in the following dilutions: weak 1 : 100,000 or medium 1 : 10,000 without effect. Some patients did show an effect after intradermal injection of a 1 : 100 or a 1 : 1000 solution. This proved that resistance toward tuberculosis is often low in hunger disease. According to Grover's classification this is called pleiosthesy and is responsible for the high incidence of tuberculous infection and its fulminating course.

We considered the possibility that the skin loses its capacity for reacting to tuberculin. The research of Dr. B. Raszkes (manuscript lost) proved that the skin of these patients demonstrated a low degree of reactivity to intradermal injections of morphine and adrenalin and a somewhat higher but still low degree of reactivity to caffeine. Reduced skin reactivity alone, however, could not entirely explain the reduced response to tuberculin since our eye specialist repeated this research using the method described by Calmet. He injected a 1 : 100 solution of tuberculin into the conjunctiva. The reaction was almost negative even without the skin's being involved.

We planned to pursue this allergenic research but were unable to for reasons beyond our control. The fact that people with hunger disease are so easily infected with tuberculosis can be explained by their general lack of resistance, and by the decreased oxygenation of the hungry tissues, slow blood circulation, hypokinemia, defective capillarization of the lungs, and hypoanergy of the organism (more about this below). These factors may also explain the severe course of tuberculosis in our patients.

The paralysis of fighting forces of the organism, its lack of energy, diminishes the tendency to develop connective tissue in the lungs and cancels the action of the immunity factors which combat contagion.

In patients with hunger disease there is a tendency toward purulent and cheesy tuberculosis not only in the lungs but also in the pleura, the skin, the intestinal lymphatic glands, and the peritoneum. Amyloidosis was rarely present in pulmonary tuberculosis or in lung abscesses. Its absence can be explained by the short duration of the disease and the undernutrition during the war years. The lack of animal protein and the resulting lack of amino acids like cystine and cysteine agree with the latest theories on the origin of amyloidosis.

Patients with hunger disease often suffer from bronchitis and from almost asymptomatic bronchopneumonia. Pseudopneumonia is sometimes really pneumomalatia, which destroys the lungs with cavitations.

Bronchial asthma and other allergic diseases are very rare; on the contrary, one sees spontaneous recovery from urticaria, hayfever, gastritis, enteritis, bronchial asthma, and food allergy. It is difficult to state whether this is due to the acidosis in hunger disease, as postulated by Tiefensee, or to hypoanergy as described by our group, manifesting itself by the weak reaction of the body toward tuberculin or pharmacological stimulants. Pneumonia with pleural effusions is connected with the tendency of the organism to retain large amounts of fluid in the Archard cavities system. Sometimes there is fluid in the peritoneal cavity, and fluid may even be present in the pericardial cavity, though this is rare.

There are many changes in the circulatory system in hunger disease. Since the metabolism in resting persons is very low we could expect reduced circulatory action. According to Terroine, the function of the circulatory system is to provide oxygen for cells and tissues and to remove carbon dioxide.

During World War I it was noted that the pulse was sometimes as low as 32 beats per minute (as a result of sinus bradycardia). There was low arterial pressure, mute heartbeats, low voltage on electrocardiographic curves, and often retarded auriculoventricular conduction.

We made the following observations. The heart is covered by the lungs. Its size and shape are normal. Heartbeats are faint and without accessory murmurs. Sometimes bellows sounds which imitate functional murmurs are heard. Heart activity is low, 40 to 50 beats per minute, and sometimes 36 to 38 per minute. Activity above 70 to 80 beats per minute is rare. Sometimes one observes pallid diffuse cyanosis like a fine net covering the nose, the cheeks, most of the legs, soles, forearms, and palms. After the blankets are removed parts of the patient become very cold, especially if the room is cold, demonstrating poor adaptation to thermal changes. The arteries in young patients are straight, narrow, flabby and hardly palpable. The antecubital veins as well as veins in other areas are hardly visible. The pulse is regular, weak, slow, synchronous with the apex beat, and not easily stimulated. The blood pressure is low—systolic 80 to 100 and sometimes as low as 60, and diastolic 50 to 60 and sometimes even 40.

We did some clinical research on the functional relationship between the circulatory system and the autonomic nervous system. Twenty patients were examined to determine the effect of body position on blood pressure and pulse rate using our "swing" method. The fasting patient is placed on a mobile operating table or rocking chair and his body position is rotated from the Trendelenburg position, 45° below horizontal, to horizontal 0°. Then the head is elevated to +45°, to +90°, and finally to vertical, +180°. Under these circumstances a normal person shows an increase in both systolic and diastolic blood pressure, and an increase in pulse rate. In cachexia or hunger edema the body scarcely reacts to these position changes and sometimes the reaction is just the opposite of normal (Figure 1).

We examined the effect of a protein load on blood pressure and pulse by using our method of feeding fasting patients four hard boiled eggs. After 2 hours normal people show increasing blood pressures and pulse rates when measured every 20 minutes. In liver disease systolic pressure becomes lower. In cachexia and hunger edema there is no reaction or a very slight lowering of blood pressure (Figure 2).

The director of our department conducted a number of studies on the function of the circulatory system. He found not only low arterial pressure but also low venous pressure (10 to 20 mm water). There was also a weak oscillometric change as

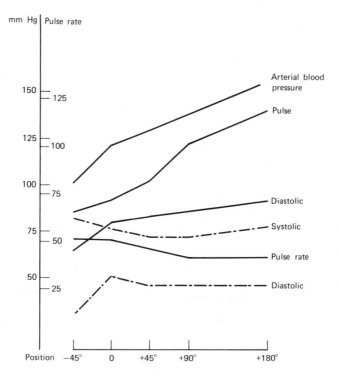

Figure 1   Swing test. Solid line: normal; dashed line: hunger disease.

measured with a Recklinhaus oscillometer. The volume of circulating blood measured by the Griesbach method with Congo red increased from 99 to 162 cc per kg of body weight. There was an increased circulation time, sometimes as much as twofold (from 40 to 80 seconds), and a slowing down of capillary circulation and concomitant diminution of the minute volume of the heart. Normal volume as measured by this method is 8 to 10 liters. In hunger disease patients the maximum was 1.5 liters. Finally, in some rare cases, systolic discharge was reduced to 15 cc; in normal subjects it is 90 to 100 cc.

Electrocardiograms revealed flat low P waves and QRS complexes as well as sinus bradycardia.

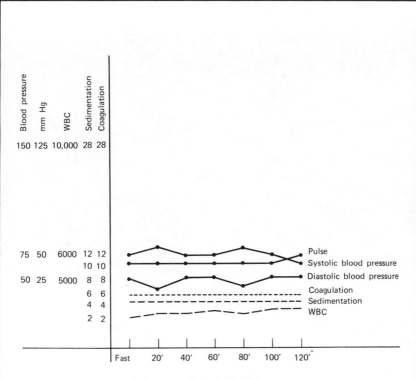

Figure 2   Hard boiled egg test.

In contrast to what occurs in normal subjects, after physical stress patients with hunger disease showed no change in venous and arterial blood pressure. After 20 situps in 20 cases there were no changes in the respiratory rate and tidal volume of the lungs. Some research was done on the effects of the autonomic nervous system on the circulation using the ocular pressure test and pharmacological stimulation with subcutaneous adrenalin (Figure 3, 40 cases), subcutaneous pilocarpine (Figure 4, 30 cases), and intravenous atropine (Figure 5, 30 cases). Pressure on the eyeballs or subcutaneous injection of adrenergic or cholinergic drugs does not affect the pulse or blood pressure. The usual effects such as salivation, sweating, tremor, changes in the pupils, or palpitations do not occur. The intravenous atropine test consisted of injecting 0.25 mg of atropine nitrate every few

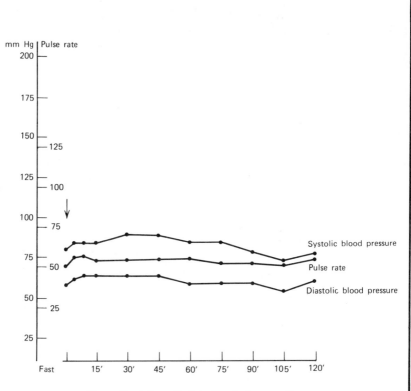

Figure 3   Adrenalin injection in hunger disease.

minutes until paralysis of the cholinergic system occurred as demonstrated by a constant pulse, even after pressing the eyeballs. The hunger disease patients had to be injected with 2.0 to 2.5 mg of atropine to demonstrate any effect. The results demonstrate diminished tension of the two antagonistic systems (hypoamphotony). When normal tension exists in the cholinergic system tension in the adrenergic system is diminished. In addition, when adrenergic tension is normal cholinergic tension is increased. To put it in other words, there always was hyperfunction of the cholinergic system even in hypoamphotony.

Clinical changes and results of research on functions of the circulatory system in cases of cachexia and hunger edema show

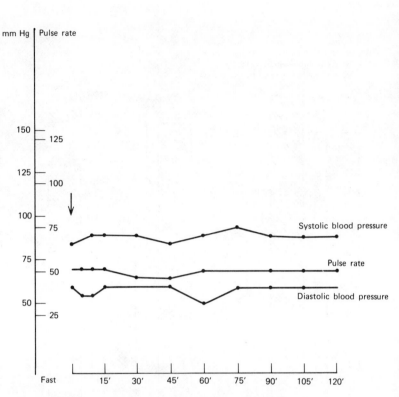

Figure 4 Pilocarpine injection in hunger disease.

definitive asthenia. Reduced cardiac output is accompanied by diminished arterial and venous pressures and is associated with impaired peripheral blood circulation. The symptoms of coldness, pallor, and peripheral cyanosis of the extremities, reduced capillary circulation, impaired thermal adaptation, weak peripheral oscillatory changes, and a tendency to frostbite even in early fall are all part of the same syndrome. Some of our patients, upon entering the ward, often look as though they are in a severe state of collapse. The pallid, cyanotic, cold extremities and almost undetectable filiform pulse are typical symptoms of collapse. In addition the weak pulse and mute heart sounds as well

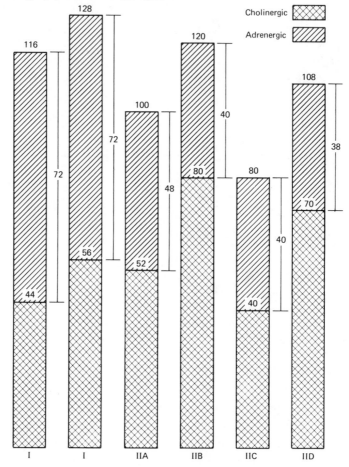

Figure 5   Eye atropine test.

as the low arterial and venous pressures confirm this diagnosis. By contrast other findings, such as increase in the volume of circulating blood and plasma, are against this diagnosis.

The following factors must be considered in explaining the disturbances in the circulation. Changes within the heart as confirmed by clinical and electrocardiographic findings contribute not only to the circulatory changes but also to the increase in circulating blood volume. The complete absence of passive congestion in the lungs, the liver, or the kidneys suggests that circulatory collapse is a protective mechanism, instrumental in preventing this passive congestion. Decreased circulation time, decrease of blood volume per minute, and decrease of systolic discharges are characteristic of cardiac and vascular insufficiency. In addition, such peripheral factors as advanced anemia and a cholinergic tendency prevent the pulse from accelerating. Characteristic for cachexia and hunger edema is the lack of circulatory or respiratory response to stimuli like changes in body posture, oral protein load, physical exertion, and certain drugs. Long lasting hunger very often eliminates tachycardia and other circulatory neuroses which existed before the war. There was no arteriosclerosis or spontaneous hypertension of second or third degree, which were quite common before the war.

The hematopoietic system was examined by our specialists. We measured bleeding and coagulation time and blood morphology. This work was also done on children. We examined blood of patients from another ward and studied bone marrow of adults and children (this work was lost).

Red blood cells examined in 80 cases decreased from 3 million per mm^3 to between 1.5 and 1 million and in some cases even below. Hemoglobin decreased to 60 to 70% and in some cases ranged as low as 10%. Color index was usually 1 or less, and rarely reached 1.15. Examining a drop of fresh blood we noticed that the red blood cells do not aggregate normally into rolls but remain single or group into small clusters. Anisocytosis and even more often microcytosis are present, macrocytosis is rare, and there are no nucleated red blood cells. Often the red blood cells are colorless and irregularly shaped. These are symptoms of hypochromic anemia in the recovery phase as indicated by a high percentage of reticulocytes (8 to 10%).

The morphological changes were influenced by the normal or increased volume of circulating blood and the reduced body weight. We had two women patients weighing about 30 kg; one had 3.5 liters of blood, the other 4.2 liters. Both were obviously cases of normovolemia or even hypervolemia. In several patients hematocrit values were determined. The normal value is about 45. In our patients values ranged from 35 to as low as 10.

In cachexia and hunger edema there is no anemia in the strict sense because blood volume is not decreased in proportion to body weight. Since there is a low percentage of red blood cells in a drop of blood, this would be classified as normovolemic oligocytemia.

We studied 40 blood samples to determine water content in undernourished patients by drying a free flowing drop from a finger and a free flowing drop of venous blood to constant weight in a vacuum desiccator and by weighing fresh samples of whole blood, red blood cells, and plasma.

In order to obtain a better constant dry weight the samples after the first weighing were hemolyzed with double distilled water, as described in our paper published from Dr. W. Orlowski's clinic. This is an accurate method of determining the water content of blood. The relationship of plasma to red blood cells was established by centrifugation at 3000 to 3500 revolutions per minute. At this speed red blood cells are not damaged. In normal specimens plasma contains 89 to 90% water and red blood cells contain 63 to 67% water. In our patients' specimens plasma contained 93 to 94% water and red blood cells only 58%.

The changes described in the water content of the blood can produce a pseudoanemia in patients with cachexia or hunger edema. The dryness of the red blood cells explains the presence of microcytosis.

The sedimentation rate does not change in our patients. An increased sedimentation rate in these patients was often the earliest and most sensitive sign of concomitant active tuberculosis.

It is a known fact that in patients with liver disease the sedimentation rate increases after meals, especially meals containing proteins. In our patients this did not occur after our hard boiled egg test.

The white blood cell count is 3000 to 4000 per mm^3. Normal counts or even levels as high as 13,000 to 14,000 per mm^3 are often seen in complications like colitis, suppurating dermatosis, or frostbite.

The hard boiled egg load did not affect the white blood cell count in 20 cases, though an occasional increase was observed. In the Vidal test even a load of a glass of milk increases the white blood cell count within 20 to 120 minutes in normal people. In patients with liver disease the white blood cell count decreases. We could not carefully examine the effect of drugs like adrenalin on the white blood cell count. However, in one experiment the injection of adrenalin resulted in a lymphocytosis rather than the expected leukocytosis.

The morphology of the white blood cell shows mostly uninuclear lymphocytes and monocytes. The percentage of lymphocytes in adults without tuberculosis can reach up to 50%. There were no eosinophiles in the peripheral blood samples although they were found in the intravital bone marrow samples. The platelet count diminished to 50,000 to 70,000 per mm^3 (manuscript lost).

Intravital samples of bone marrow are full of cellular elements. Bleeding and coagulation time were usually normal and only occasionally was the coagulation time accelerated.

There was no positive Rumpel-Leede sign in the clinical picture of diathesis.

We have already discussed the changes in the oral cavity caused by starvation. A lowering of the intestines (Glenard's disease) connected with the terrible body weight loss was very commonly observed. X-rays of clinic patients with nonspecific complaints show atony of the stomach without any change in its position.

In 20 cases we measured the stomach acidity 10 times after an alcohol load and 10 times after a caffein load. Similar work was done on children in the Children's Hospital. No hyperacidity was found. The values of general acidity and free hydrochloric acid were low, 8 to 10, and sometimes in cases of hunger edema there was complete achylia (no total or free acid).

Duodenal or stomach ulcers, gastritis, and ileitis were all rare. To explain the lack of these symptoms one must consider many factors. For example, low acidity and lowered susceptibility toward allergens, mostly from food, could be due in part to the completely changed diet, which is lacking in fat and hence in its degradation products like volatile fatty acids, and which contains large amounts of cellulose, which speeds the passing of food through the gastrointestinal tract. The degree of stomach acidity and the rarity of ulcers can be connected to the lack of hydrochloric acid or allergic reactions. It is interesting that the vagus nerve is so highly active in the circulatory system and has such low activity as to be almost paralyzed in the functions of the stomach. As for the intestines, we must emphasize a different ailment connected with the faulty diet—increased peristalsis, drumbelly, and very copious bowel movements. Enteritis, with bloody and mucous bowel movements, is a very common complication of long term hunger; it increases hunger edema and accelerates death.

Increased loss of protein through the digestive system is also responsible for these symptoms. Atonic rectum is obvious upon rectal examination. Undernourished patients seldom suffer from liver or gall bladder ailments. When these diseases do exist, the patients adjust well to hunger. Sometimes they feel much better than before the war, when they were not able to work. Gall bladder function was studied by introducing Einhorn's catheter into the duodenum and trying to induce the Meltzer Lyon reflex, the emptying of the contents of the gall bladder into the intestine. Our findings were:

1. The first portion of the duodenal content is very pale, almost colorless.

2. The usual stimuli, such as a solution of magnesium sulfate, are not enough to obtain samples of bile. For that result pituitrin had to be used.
3. The Meltzer Lyon reflex is very slow.

Obviously the gall bladder is suffering from atony (cholecysto-atony). For technical reasons we could not confirm these findings by cholecystography. Several times we detected the presence of *Lambia intestinalis* in the gall bladder contents.

One of the best methods for determining liver function is the honey load effect on blood coagulation and the extent of uro-bilinogenuria and the changes in the blood sugar curve after a levulose load. The levulose load test was technically impossible to conduct, and the results would be uncertain anyway because of the abnormal long term diet of people with hunger disease.

We were able to use our method of hard boiled egg load on 20 patients. The following observations were made:

1. Within 2 to 3 hours after the load urobilinogenuria appears.
2. Within 20 to 120 minutes there is lowering of white blood cell count.
3. Within 20 to 120 minutes there is a decrease in blood pressure.
4. Sedimentation time increased.
5. Blood coagulation is enhanced.

We detected 14 cases of urobilinogenuria in 20 examined samples. Our test discovers latent dysfunction of the liver by breaking the liver barrier with the load of protein and cholesterol —the two nutrients missing for so long in the war diet.

As for the pancreas, feces examination in several cases detected food that ordinarily could have been digested. There was a large quantity of vegetal cellulose, and debris resembling oats was visible on gross inspection. Diastase in urine was determined in 20 patients. The fluctuations did not exceed the limitations of the methods; therefore we assume that pancreatic function in hunger disease is not damaged.

Some general practitioners without examining the urine would send patients with hunger edema to the hospital, suspecting kidney disease. Our findings on renal function revealed:

1. Normal urine analysis.
2. Low blood pressure.
3. Small heart size (microcardia).
4. No changes in the eye fundus.
5. Low blood urea (sometimes below the normal level).

Concentrating ability and the response to an oral water load was tested in 20 patients. Concentrating ability is often inadequate, reaching only 1015, whereas diluting capacity is normal, reaching 1002 to 1001. The water load is eliminated within 4 hours. Sometimes an even larger volume was excreted than the volume ingested. The patients with hunger edema would lose up to 1 kg of body water in 4 hours. This demonstrates negative water balance and enhanced ability of the kidneys to eliminate water. These findings help explain the role of subcutaneous tissue in the development of hunger edema. There is accelerated absorption of intradermally injected saline solution in cachexia and hunger edema.

With regard to the bones and joints, there is a tendency to osteomalacia, spontaneous breaks of the neck of the femur in young people, and slow healing of spontaneous breaks. Surgeons were reluctant to implant metal pins in breaks because the bone tissue was often thin and soft. Unfortunately we could not document our findings with appropriate X-rays.

The neuromuscular system was studied but the manuscripts were lost. Reflexes such as chin hand, chin lips, Babinski's, and Chvostek's were often abnormal. There were many signs of supersensitivity of the neuromuscular system, such as reflex contraction of the muscles of the chest after pinching the skin or striking it with a reflex hammer. There were cases of typical muscle spasms in adults or growing youths, mostly in the springtime, or spasmodic syndromes after injections of salirgan. According to the reports from the neurology wards and clinics

TABLE 1 DEATH RATE AMONG THE JEWISH POPULATION
IN WARSAW DURING THE WAR

Month and Year	Typhus (Reported Cases)	Total Deaths from All Causes	Death Typhus	Death Hunger	Death Unknown
September 1939	—	1,936	—	—	650
October 1939	—	1,850	—	—	744
November 1939	—	1,595	—	1	411
December 1939	—	1,179	5	3	251
Total	—	6,560	5	4	2,056
January 1940	95	1,178	17	16	140
February 1940	206	1,179	26	25	192
March 1940	392	1,014	34	14	126
April 1940	403	1,044	57	13	187
May 1940	350	856	47	5	63
June 1940	122	650	17	1	60
July 1940	67	563	10	2	35
August 1940	18	525	1	—	32
September 1940	18	489	1	2	68
October 1940	16	457	—	1	47
November 1940	23	445	3	3	25
December 1940	17	581	3	9	57
Total	1,727	8,981	216	91	1,032
January 1941	57	898	4	81	93
February 1941	129	1,023	14	120	77
March 1941	201	1,608	23	264	125
April 1941	241	2,061	21	490	206
May 1941	367	3,821	38	1,349	738
June 1941	841	4,590	89	1,599	824
July 1941	1,742	5,550	246	1,419	1,436
August 1941	1,805	5,560	226	1,376	1,530
September 1941	2,492	4,545	272	889	1,553
October 1941	3,438	4,716	472	1,033	1,267
November 1941	2,156	4,801	309	1,188	1,476
December 1941	1,980	4,366	277	1,163	1,328
Total	15,449	43,239	1,991	10,971	10,653
January 1942	1,220	5,123	220	1,712	1,563
February 1942	787	4,618	119	1,495	1,680
March 1942	478	4,951	80	1,385	2,132
April 1942	319	4,432	46	935	2,354
May 1942	208	3,636	36	880	1,642
June 1942	118	3,356	11	847	1,323
July 1942	67	3,672	—	—	—
August 1942	—	4,516	—	—	—
September 1942	—	4,244	—	—	—
October 1942	6	423	—	—	—
November 1942	20	414	—	—	—
December 1942					
Total	3,223	39,385	512	7,254	10,694

there were many cases of polyneuritis. We have already mentioned the contractures of the extremities, which were often present.

The most striking psychiatric finding is the prevalence of depression, even in young people. There is complete apathy, lack of interest, poor thinking, and even incoherence.

Infectious diseases such as typhus, diphtheria, diffuse abscesses, erysipelas, and virulent tuberculosis were extremely common. By contrast, tonsillitis, scarlet fever, rheumatism, and meningitis were rare.

Changes in metabolism and endocrine glands will be described in Chapter 3.

Persistent hunger results in very pronounced weight loss. Devoid of subcutaneous fat, boys and girls from blooming like roses change into withered old people. One of the patients said, "Our strength is vanishing like a melting wax candle." Active, busy, energetic people are changed into apathetic, sleepy beings, always in bed, hardly able to get up to eat or to go to the toilet. Passage from life to death is slow and gradual, like death from physiological old age. There is nothing violent, no dyspnea, no pain, no obvious changes in breathing or circulation. Vital functions subside simultaneously. Pulse rate and respiratory rate get slower and it becomes more and more difficult to reach the patient's awareness, until life is gone. People fall asleep in bed or on the street and are dead in the morning. They die during physical effort, such as searching for food, and sometimes even with a piece of bread in their hands. Included in Table 1, prepared by the Jewish Council, are statistics on the various causes of death. The category "unknown" usually means hunger.

EDITOR'S COMMENTS

Myron Winick, M.D.

The clinical picture of hunger disease as seen in the patients from the Warsaw ghetto begins with a description of their diet. Officially, these people were permitted 800 calories per day, consisting of about 3 g of fat (less than 5% of calories), 20 to 30 g of vegetable protein (10 to 15% of calories), and the rest (more than 80%) carbohydrate. The protein was of very low quality and the food was deficient in certain vitamins and minerals, particularly fat soluble vitamins A, D, K, and E, calcium, and iron. The population, although carefully selected, varied in the exact nature of their diets. Some consumed even less than the "permitted" amount of 800 calories, while others managed to supplement this diet with food smuggled into the ghetto.

With this pattern of food consumption the initial complaints were frequently thirst, polyuria and nocturia, dryness of the mouth, rapid weight loss, and a constant craving for food. Many of these findings had been described before and were noted and carefully documented subsequently in the extensive studies carried out in the late 1940s by Keys and his co-workers in Minnesota. A complete review of the various clinical observations in semi-starvation, including the findings in the studies from the Warsaw ghetto of which they became aware long after their own studies were in progress, is reported in their book published in 1950. Because of the proximity in time of the two studies (the Warsaw study preceding those in Minnesota by about five years) comparisons will undoubtedly be made. Many observations were similar, others were different, and I do not intend to make detailed comparisons. The two studies were designed quite differently and hence ask somewhat different questions. However, they complement each other extremely well and together paint a much more complete picture of semistarvation than either study alone. The study by Keys and co-workers was longitudinal and hence the authors could observe serial changes. The patients were all rehabilitated and observations could be made during the recovery period. Again serial changes could be noted. The Warsaw ghetto study was by necessity cross sectional. The degree of starvation was greater and its duration much longer. In addition, the patients rarely recovered, most progressing to death. Those that did recover did so spontaneously, without a major change in diet. Therefore the authors of the Warsaw studies were able to describe in detail progressive starvation unto death. At no time previously nor at any time since have such detailed observations of this nature been made.

They describe weight loss which reached 50% of prewar weight in many of their patients, and divide hunger into three degrees:

1. Depletion of fat reserves.
2. Aging and withering of the patient.
3. Terminal cachexia.

Most of the patients were already in the second phase. The careful description of "premature aging" extends to various organs and, as we shall see, the changes are most drastic in the eye and in the skeletal system.

Observations on the pigmentation of the skin and its pale, dry, scaly condition were not new. However the conclusion that the pigmentation occurred in traumatized areas was new. In addition, the dirty brown pigmentation of the face and in some cases the conjunctiva and the tongue in the last stages of the disease was first described in this study. They also noted the extreme ease with which the skin could be traumatized. Finally, a widespread sensitivity of the skin to the rays of the sun, especially in the spring, is noted. Patients often experienced redness, swelling, local hyperthermia, and fever blisters after only one exposure. Abnormal hair growth is carefully noted, luxuriant if hunger occurred during puberty, but with alopecia if it occurred later. Hair was extremely brittle, thick, and uneven.

The description of the edema of hunger disease is extremely detailed and some of the observations were unique at the time. For example, these investigators point out that water absorption from the skin was increased, and actually quantitated this by performing the Aldrich-McClure test in which a water blister is introduced under the skin. Normally it takes 60 minutes for this blister to disappear; in these patients it disappeared in 20 to 30 minutes.

As many investigators had noted before and have described subsequently, general hypothermia was present. What is more interesting is the observation made here that the temperature response to diseases which usually produce a high fever, such as typhus, was blunted.

Examination of the musculature demonstrated marked atrophy and generalized weakness. In addition, creatine was measurable in the urine in 17 out of 20 patients, suggesting active muscle breakdown. Again, this observation of demonstrable creatinuria was original with these investigators.

The eye changes are documented in greater detail in a subsequent chapter. However in this chapter certain very important clinical observations are made. Thin conjunctiva, which are often spotted with brown, blue sclerae, and the absence of Bitot spots, corneal softening, or night blindness were noted. This last is an important observation because it essentially rules out vitamin A deficiency as a major contributor to the clinical manifestations of hunger disease as seen in the Warsaw ghetto. This is interesting in view of the diet, which must have been low in vitamin A, and raises the question whether this population, which was reasonably well nourished before the war, had sufficient vitamin A reserves to prevent frank deficiency even when exposed to a low intake of vitamin A for a relatively long time. These observations also must make us re-evaluate the dry, scaly, desquamating skin that was almost universally observed. The etiology of these changes was not likely to have been vitamin A deficiency. Perhaps the low fat diet (less than 5% of calories as total fat) dropped the linoleic acid content below 1% of calories and the skin manifestations were those of essential fatty acid deficiency, a disease which was not adequately appreciated at that time. Perhaps the skin changes were those of prolonged exposure to reduced calories in general. We can only speculate at this point but my own interpretation would be that essential fatty acid deficiency was prevalent and was a major contributor to the skin manifestations.

Other changes in the eye also give a better general picture of severe hunger disease. Premature cataracts were observed and careful observations revealed them to be indistinguishable from senile cataracts. This lends strong support to the author's thesis that premature aging is an important component of the overall picture of hunger disease. The mechanism by which this acceleration of aging might occur is unknown and certainly, if it exists, represents a challenge not only to those interested in the effects of starvation but also to those interested in the process of aging.

The author notes a number of changes in the oral cavity, none of which is specific for hunger disease. The high prevalence of dental caries noted, for example, is probably due to poor oral hygiene. A very interesting observation is the change in the voice that occurred in patients in the terminal phase of hunger disease. He describes it as extremely hoarse *vox cholerica,* and is uncertain whether this change was due to a functional paralysis of the vocal cords or to generalized tissue dehydration.

A new syndrome is described by the author. He notes radiolucent lungs, free costophrenic angles, a lowering of the lung borders, and decreased pulmonary mobility, all in the absence of any tubercular signs. He ascribes these findings to long term hunger alone and speculates that these pulmonary changes and poor ventilation create conditions which increase the incidence of active tuberculosis.

In relation to tuberculosis these investigators made a very important observation concerning the reaction to tuberculin. Even patients with active tuberculosis often did not react to intradermal injection of tuberculin. The author ascribed this either to poor reactivity of the skin or to a poor allergic response. The lack of response to tuberclin on the conjunctiva suggested the latter. Today we have learned a great deal about this lack of response. It constitutes a reduced response by those factors involved in cellular immunity. The atrophied thymus and tonsils noted by these investigators is also part of this overall reduced immune response. In addition, the author notes not only that certain typical allergic diseases, such as bronchial asthma, urticaria, hayfever, and food allergies, occurred rarely, but that patients who were suffering from these illnesses for long periods of time recovered "spontaneously."

In examining the circulatory system the investigators made a number of observations which were standard by that time: bradycardia, low blood pressure, weak muffled heart sounds, straight arteries, and collapsed veins. In addition, they attempted to assess the response of the circulatory system to a defined stress—a measurable change in position. By means of a swinging table or rocking chair, body position was rotated through 180°. Under normal circumstances, systolic and diastolic blood pressure increases, as does the pulse rate. In patients with hunger disease there was usually no response, and occasionally the response was reversed. A second type of stress was introduced by giving the patient a protein load in the form of four hard boiled eggs. In normal patients, blood pressure and pulse rate increase within 2 hours. In patients with hunger disease there again is usually no response or occasionally a slight lowering of pressure and pulse.

A number of very precise observations and measurements were made on the circulatory system and these are carefully described in a subsequent chapter. The results are summarized here and demonstrate a low arterial pressure, a low venous pressure, reduced pulse pressure, increased blood volume, increased circulation time, slowing of capillary circulation, and a reduced minute volume of the heart. The responses of all of these parameters to stress and drugs were also studied. The observations will be discussed in my comments on Chapter 4, which deals with the circulatory system, but it is appropriate to point out here how well the clinical observations in this study were coordinated with the physiological studies. Obviously a "tight" protocol was maintained, with one group of investigators quite cognizant of what other groups were doing. In addition, the clinical findings are explained in physiological terms based on actual physiological measurements. Thus the author concludes that "the symptoms of coldness, pallor, and peripheral cyanosis of the extremities, reduced capillary circulation, impaired thermal adaptation, weak peripheral pulses, and a tendency to frostbite even in early fall are all part of the same syndrome."

Another interesting observation made by these investigators in relation to the circulatory system was that certain conditions improve. For example, various types of tachycardias, atherosclerosis, and spontaneous hypertension were no longer seen, although they had been very common before the war.

Very detailed hematologic studies were made by these investigators and are discussed in Chapter 5. In Chapter 1 the author notes the anemia and leukopenia as well as the reticulocytosis in some of the patients.

Studies on gastric acidity were performed both in the fasting state and after ingestion of a gastric stimulus. Almost total achlorhydria was observed in both situations. This observation was documented in both adults and children and represents the most extensive study of gastric acidity in hunger disease performed to that time. The lack of free acid in the stomach may partly explain another important observation made by these investigators—a marked decrease in the incidence of gastric and duodenal ulcers. The incidence of gastritis and ileitis also decreased, as did liver and gall bladder disease. By contrast, enteritis with bloody mucous stools was a very common complication of hunger disease. Many patients had atony of the rectal sphincter.

Special studies were carried out to investigate gall bladder function. At rest very little bile is secreted. After the usual stimuli, for example, magnesium sulfate, there was almost no response. However, with pituitrin a mild response could be elicited. The studies demonstrated relative hypotony of the gall bladder and even though they could not be confirmed radiographically they represent extremely detailed observations which again were much more complete than any previous studies.

Liver function was examined by several methods available to the investigators. These studies could not be completed, but from what they observed they concluded that latent liver dysfunction was present. Today, as a result of many studies which have been carried out on both children and adults, we are better able to understand this liver dysfunction. The synthesis of certain proteins, such as albumin and β lipoproteins, is markedly reduced. This leads to the hypoalbuminemia and fatty infiltration of the liver seen in many patients suffering from semistarvation. By contrast, other proteins, such as gamma globulins, seem to be synthesized normally. The reason for this differential liver protein synthesis still remains obscure.

On the basis of normal diastase levels in urine the author concludes that pancreatic function is normal in hunger disease. This is surprising since he carefully notes undigested food in the stool. In this situation the investigators allowed the evidence of a crude biochemical test to outweigh that of their clinical observations. As is often the case in medicine, the clinical observations were correct and today we know that pancreatic function can be severely compromised in patients with semistarvation.

The lack of concentrating ability of the kidney is carefully noted and the author points out that even in very edematous patients water balance was negative and the kidney was perfectly able to excrete copious amounts of dilute urine.

The bones are reported to show signs of advanced osteomalacia and to undergo spontaneous fractures. Healing of fractures was extremely slow and the surgeons were reluctant to insert metal pins because of the thinness of the bone tissue. Unfortunately the extent of these changes could not be documented by X-ray studies. It is difficult to ascribe these changes to a reduced intake of vitamin D, since frank rickets was not observed in the children. The markedly reduced calcium intake might be partly responsible for the bone changes. The changes described in bone are consistent with the author's theory of premature aging in hunger disease.

Unfortunately the manuscript describing the changes in the neuromuscular system was lost. However the author does comment on the frequency of muscle spasms, the large number of cases of polyneuritis, and the contractures of the extremities.

Like children, adults were extremely susceptible to certain types of infections. Typhus, diphtheria, diffuse abscesses, erysipelas, and virulent tuberculosis were extremely common. By contrast, tonsillitis, scarlet fever, rheumatic fever, and bacterial meningitis were quite rare.

The description of the final phases of hunger disease is particularly worth noting, since very few observations of this sort have been made. Gradually youth was drained and young people changed into withered old people. "Strength vanished like a melting wax candle." Severe apathy sets in and patients lie quietly in bed not sitting up even to eat or to go to the toilet. "Passage from life to death is gradual, like death from physiological old age." Pulse rate and respiratory rate drop and the patient becomes more and more stuporous until all life is gone.

After reading this chapter one can only be struck by the careful day to day, hour to hour observations that were made. But what to me is much more striking is the ability of the investigators to sustain their work. These were not investigators who came in, did their tests, and went home. These were physicians, dealing with the easiest disease to cure, and helpless to effect that cure. They cared for their patients in whatever manner they had available and at the same time carefully noted their deterioration. Afflicted with the same disease, knowing that their time was limited, they persevered. Their observations should allow us to learn a great deal and perhaps to render better care to the sick, but perhaps the best legacy they leave is their courage, their devotion to medicine, and their personal example of what the Hippocratic oath really means.

TWO   Clinical Aspects of Hunger Disease in Children

Dr. Anna Braude-Heller
Dr. Israel Rotbalsam
Dr. Regina Elbinger

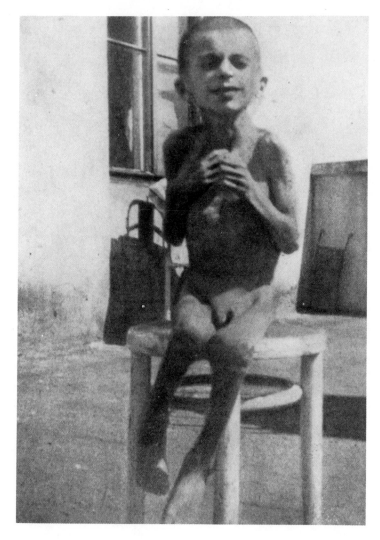

Severe muscle wasting and contractures of the flexor muscles.

The first victims of the hunger catastrophe among the Jewish population during World War II were children. In the first three years we saw several hundred children from a few months to 14 years old, who were brought to our hospital. At the end of 1939 and the beginning of 1940, we saw mostly infants. The short period of real hunger during the siege of Warsaw resulted in severe malnutrition of infants, with symptoms of dystrophy or more advanced atrophy. Edema was a rarity during this period.

The first great influx of patients was connected with the deportation of hundreds of people from small towns to Warsaw at the end of 1940. The Jewish population was locked into a ghetto, with an almost nonexistent official food supply, and the result was a terrible increase in hunger and disease. The children brought to the hospital at the end of 1940 and the beginning of 1941 were two to five years old. The youngest children showed the earliest and most pronounced hunger symptoms. Later the older children started to come to the hospital. By the time the older ones became sick, the little ones were already dead. At the end of 1941 and the beginning of 1942, most of the children we saw were over five years old. Later in 1942 we seldom saw children under eight years old. During this period we saw many terminal hunger atrophy cases without edema, and we called this form "desiccated destruction."

It was difficult to collect information from these children. Most of them were on rations from deportation centers. In the best circumstances they subsisted on 800 calories, devoid of fat and containing a minimal amount of strictly vegetable protein.

The earliest changes were psychological and behavioral. Apathy increased with the progress of the disease. The children became humorless, they stopped playing, their movements slowed down, and they were quarrelsome and bad tempered. Behavior seemed adult, but intellectual level was very low and they often seemed retarded. After the symptoms of malnutrition disappeared the psychological development regained its normal level.

In more advanced hunger the children did not get up. They lay on their sides, legs curled under. The children's ward was very typical, with the curled up immobile forms covered all the way up at night even in summer, but not sleeping—for sometimes they suffered from insomnia. In advanced cases the children were unable to get up and walk by themselves.

The primary symptom of hunger disease is loss of weight. In children with edema this loss is not so obvious, but in so-called "dry atrophy" or after the disappearance of edema, the weight lost can reach 50% of normal weight. Since growth was inhibited, the actual weight was expressed in relation to both the height and the age of the children. The stunted growth was not as terrible as the weight loss but was most striking in children when the period of hunger coincided with the period of maximal growth. Children between two and five and those between seven and nine were most afflicted. Often we saw children three to four years old no bigger than infants, or nine year olds looking like five or six year olds at most. The children exposed to hunger just before the onset of puberty looked rather tall because they were so thin, but their growth was not so stunted as that of younger children.

Body temperature was usually low. Even in infectious diseases such as measles, diphtheria, or chicken pox the temperature was only mildly elevated. We saw many cases of tuberculosis, some with severe symptoms, but the temperature was normal or even below normal.

Skin symptoms were numerous. The color was usually pale, depending on blood supply and presence of edema. Many children had cyanosis and cold palms and soles. Most children had highly pigmented brown spots, large and small, often connecting with each other. Pigmentation was localized mainly around old scars, and on the back, neck, and belly, where there was close contact between clothing and skin. Sometimes the skin was uniformly brown. These symptoms were visible in children above five years. They were more pronounced in children without edema. Besides pigmentation, we observed increased hair growth around the neck and on the cheeks. The skin was very

dry, with characteristic flaky desquamations in different degrees of intensity. In cases of terminal cachexia skinfolds took a long time to unfold. This symptom, prevalent among atrophic infants, was noticeable in young children even with advanced edema.

The localization and extent of edema depended on the age of the child. Infants and children up to two years old seldom were edematous. Edema was most often present at two to five years. After five years most children were cachexic. Edema would appear first on the face and the feet, and in small children it would quickly cover the entire body. In older children this process was somewhat slower. Edema was symmetrical, with the lower part of the body more afflicted. Persistent one-sided edema would lead to suspicion of a bloodclot in the pelvic or femoral vein. This complication was quite common, and autopsy would show advanced tuberculosis. In generalized edema there were usually pleural effusions, ascites, pericardial effusions, and fluid in the scrotum and labia majora.

The Aldrich-McClure skin water test was tried on 30 children. Disappearance time was usually accelerated even after edema subsided, which was confirmed on repeating the test on the same child. Normal test time is 45 minutes. In our patients it was 5 to 13 minutes. In dry atrophy (cachexia) the blister would last a little longer—17 to 23 minutes—but still for a shorter time than normal.

The skin was very easily infected with impetigo, erythema, cheilitis, and parasitic conditions such as scabies, fungi, and lice, which led to inflammatory symptoms. The reactions of the skin to chemical stimuli or antigens were weak. Dr. B. Raszkes, our colleague, studied our patients, injecting different chemical and pharmaceutical substances intradermally, and he was able to demonstrate diminished reactivity of the skin. (His manuscript was lost.)

In everyday clinical observation the lack of a positive tuberculin reaction was striking. Pigment reaction was usually negative, even in completely proven cases of tuberculosis. Intradermal reaction to a 1 : 1000 Mantoux test was negative. Even a 1 : 100 solution did not always give a positive reaction. A positive reaction usually occurs in cases where tuberculosis is localized in focal infiltrations or affects peripheral glands. The lack of a positive Mantoux test in cases of proven tuberculosis demonstrates that skin has a selective anergy toward tuberculin in cases of hunger disease.

Subcutaneous tissue was always atrophied. It consisted of a very thin layer with characteristic fatty clumps the size of a grain of millet.

Lymphatic peripheral glands were palpable, hard, and movable, and showed signs of micropoliadeny. Enlargement of these glands would be expected, given the frequent inflammatory changes in the skin. The glands were also more prominent because of the atrophy of surrounding subcutaneous tissue. A characteristic sign in most terminally ill children was enlargement of the parotid and submaxillary glands. Parotids were protruding visibly, although they were not painful at palpation. The apertures of Stenson's ducts were normal. The sublingual salivary glands were not enlarged and produced very little saliva. Probably the edema of the glands was more visible because of the atrophy of surrounding fatty tissue.

Muscle strength was considerably reduced and muscle atrophy was advanced to the point that skin was just adhering to the bones. Children not disfigured by edema looked like skeletons covered with skin. The long bones, with ectasia of epiphyses, showed certain aspects of rickets, but careful measurements and X-ray findings did not substantiate this diagnosis. In many children we observed definite large separations in straight abdominal muscles.

Muscle contractures were associated mainly with long lasting hunger atrophy and affected first the flexors of the shins and the thighs and to a lesser extent the flexors of the forearms. The reason for the contractures was the long stay in a coiled position without any active motion. The formation of these contractures was prompted by muscular atrophy and probably by biochemical changes in the muscle fibers. Active and passive movements of the hip joints, the knee, and to a lesser degree the elbow were limited, but we did not notice joint ankylosis. The contractures disappeared very slowly; they persisted for a long time even after the child started regaining strength, and prevented him from walking. The children looked very peculiar with bent knees, adducted thighs, and compensating kyphosis of the lumbar portion. When the children regained strength their walk was still "ducklike" in spite of normal X-rays of the axis of the femoral column and the shaft of the femur made in the erect and recumbent positions. This waddling walk was obviously the result of atony of muscles and ligaments.

The bones were perfectly normal. Our observations of rickets are interesting. We saw rickets very rarely during the war. Only in the last year, with the new influx of refugees, did rachitic tissue appear in infants and two year old toddlers. We did not see rickets in children above two years old.

The X-ray findings in the long bones were normal. In a few cases there were signs of decalcification, but lines of growth and the shape of the bones were not changed. This paradoxical situation is the opposite of what was found during World War I, where even older children and teenagers suffered from *rachitis tarda*. In addition to the fact that very few infants survived, the children admitted to the hospital or being examined in the clinics were immediately given vitamin D as a prevention, a treatment which was not yet used during World War I. The diet is the most important factor in the pathogenesis of rickets. We will discuss this subject when speaking in general about pathogenesis of hunger symptoms. The same observations concern scurvy in hunger disease. There were none of the periostial effusions so characteristic of scurvy, no changes in muscles, skin, or oral cavity. The inflamed gums that we noticed occasionally were the result of poor or nonexistent oral or dental hygiene. On the other hand, common symptoms were smooth tongue, small tonsils, and atrophy of the lymphatic system of the oral cavity.

The first symptoms of hunger disease in the respiratory system were emphysema, lowering of the lung borders, diminished respiratory mobility, hypokinesis, tympanic resonance, and decreased breath sounds. In a few cases we observed the characteristic rounding of the chest cavity seen in severe emphysema. All these symptoms result from the same atrophic processes observed in other organs. Twice, in addition to all these symptoms, we witnessed attacks of dyspnea, similar to asthma. The general breathing was often shallow but regular.

Children with advanced edema had pleural effusions which at the onset appeared on one side only because the children always lay on one side. In diagnosing pleural effusions we had to be cautious, because often there was specific pleurisy with tubercular changes in the lungs. The differential diagnosis was very difficult because tuberculin tests were negative and there was no fever. After being surprised a few times during autopsies, we decided to tap each child with pleural effusions for diagnostic purposes. The following case history illustrates the diagnostic difficulties. An 11 year old child was admitted to the hospital with diarrhea lasting on and off for several months and edema which appeared a few weeks before the hospital admission. On examination we found advanced atrophy, general edema, ascites, and a right pleural effusion. Tuberculin reaction was negative; there was no fever; X-ray showed complete infiltration of the pleura, but pleural tapping on two occasions yielded no fluid. During the hospital stay the diarrhea subsided but the child's constitution worsened and the edema increased. Since the kidneys and the circulatory system were normal we decided that hunger disease was the cause of the edema. Autopsy revealed extensive calcification of the right pleura, cavitating tuberculosis in the right apex, some inflammatory liquid in the left pleura, tuberculosis of the peritoneal mesenteric glands, inflammatory fluid in the peritoneal cavity, and tubercular ulcerations of the intestines. Such surprising autopsies were not rare.

In the circulatory system most changes occurred in peripheral vessels. The pulse was slower than normal—in a five to six year old 50 to 60 beats a minute is considered bradycardia because a child's pulse is faster than an adult's. The blood pressure was low—systolic 60 to 65 mm Hg is indeed very low even for children. Long lasting low pulse pressure was a bad sign. Often children had a normal heartbeat and almost no detectable pulse.

Hunger Disease

When we add to these symptoms vasorelaxation, tendency toward formation of blood clots, cyanosis, and cold extremities, we must conclude that venal collapse is one of the features of hunger disease. In several children we observed symptoms that suggested damaged cardiac muscle—extra systole, and arrhythmias that were almost fibrillation. Unfortunately we had no facilities to take electrocardiograms.

The hematologic studies were performed on our patients by Dr. Goliborska, Dr. Kocen, and F. Ferszt. We would like to note some of their general findings.

Anemia was usually mild (3 to 3.5 million red blood cells, but sometimes under 2 million, or color index about 1). Even in advanced anemia no young red blood cells were found. In evaluating the degree of anemia, we had to consider "blood dilution," which was present in every case of severe malnutrition, even the dry form without edema. (Research was done on this subject by Dr. Goliborska and F. Ferszt.) Dr. Apfelbaum's research on the volume of blood in adults suffering from hunger disease has demonstrated an increase in blood volume per kilogram of body weight. This factor must also be considered in evaluating the degree of anemia. The white blood cell count was 5000 to 7000, with a mild lymphocytosis and a shift to the right. Very few acidophils were present, and children with severe infestations of gastrointestinal parasites had no eosinophils in their blood. The platelet count and bleeding and coagulation times were normal. We did not notice any bleeding diathesis, and Rumpel-Leede sign was usually negative. The lack of bleeding diathesis is characteristic of hunger disease in contrast to cachexia resulting from long lasting severe infections such as pleural abscesses, purulent middle ear infections in infants, typhus, or dysentery. In those infections bleeding diathesis, expressed by petechiae in skin and mucosa, is a very dangerous sign.

Peritoneal effusion was often connected with the generalized edema so typical of hunger disease. In these patients the differential diagnosis to exclude tuberculosis was even more difficult than in patients whose effusions were confined to the pleural cavity. It was important for diagnostic purposes to examine the epigastric superficial veins. In tuberculosis of the abdominal cavity, the enlarged cheesy extraperitoneal glands were pressing on the veins of the abdominal cavity and, as a result, a net of the dilated veins would appear in the hypogastrium. Often the presence of blood clots in the iliac and femoral veins was another sign of tuberculosis. Therefore, small amounts of liquid in the abdominal cavity, and dilated veins on the hypogastrium would suggest tubercular effusions.

The most prominent general gastrointestinal symptom of hunger disease was diarrhea. It could begin at any time, even at the onset of hunger disease before edema, and it sometimes persisted for the patient's entire hospital stay, terminating in death. The stools were semiliquid and muddled. Some of the children were simultaneously suffering from infections, and their stools gave the appearance of bloody colitis. We had no facilities for examining all the stools bacteriologically, but unfortunately many autopsies confirmed bloody dysentary. In a patient with known tubercular disease, diarrhea could be a symptom of intestinal tuberculosis. Some examinations for bacilli Koch, which we tried to do routinely, confirmed the diagnosis of tuberculosis.

The gastric contents of 15 children were examined after an alcohol load. After fasting, the small amount of gastric content was devoid of hydrochloric acid. After ingestion of 200 cc of 5% ethyl alcohol general acidity at the peak of digestion was 10 to 20 ml, with free HCl not above 10 ml.

The urological system was normal. Urine volume was normal, even when severe edema was present, and no pathological elements were found in urine.

Renal dilution and concentration tests were done in 25 children with a 500 to 800 cc load. The excreted water in most cases exceeded the amount found in healthy children under the same load conditions. However, excretion of water was slow in most cases, peaking 2 hours after the load was administered. These results suggest slow circulation in the tissues. Renal dilution capacity was normal, whereas the ability to concentrate was obviously damaged.

The nervous system was not damaged. There was no inflammation of peripheral nerves. Quite often tendon reflexes were symmetrically weakened. No motor or movement abnormalities were observed. Ten children demonstrated lower than normal nervous excitability to galvanic stimulation. In two cases with severe edema, the administration of a diuretic containing mercury resulted in intensive diuresis accompanied by typical signs of tetany. In spite of the fact that the calcium levels in the blood were normal, we assume that tetany was a symptom of disturbed mineral metabolism resulting from the intensive diuresis.

No effect was observed after the administration of adrenalin and pilocarpine. Neither of these drugs affected the pulse or the blood pressure except in a very minor way. There was little increase in sweating or salivation, and pupils were not significantly dilated. These symptoms indicate a reduced excitability of the autonomic system. However, symptoms like bradycardia, low blood pressure, and respiratory arrhythmia suggest that both the sympathetic and parasympathetic components of the vagus system are affected.

Children reaching puberty showed underdevelopment of the sex organs and lack of hair in the genital regions. Girls did not menstruate and their breasts were poorly developed.

Finally we shall discuss how children with hunger disease reacted toward infections. There is no doubt that a malnourished organism succumbs easily to tuberculosis. Tuberculosis was prevalent among our children and caused great diagnostic problems. A separate chapter in this book deals with tuberculosis (manuscript lost). Here we will mention only that we observed many serious forms of the disease, with effusions and caseation predominating. The active proliferative processes were somewhat inhibited. Besides tuberculosis of the lungs, we saw many cases of tuberculosis of the intestines and peritoneal glands, which might also be attributed to the terrible sanitary conditions. Toward the end, in 1942, we saw tuberculosis of the brain, and very rarely (in two girls, 10 and 12 years old) tuberculosis of the sex organs.

The acute and violent course, the vast changes in loco of the primary infection, the tendency to decomposition, and the lack of active processes were similar to infantile tuberculosis rather than the cavitating tuberculosis of adults. This course shows the lack of defenses of the organism toward the tuberculosis bacillus.

The response of the organism to acute infections was quite different. People cooped together and not moving much from place to place were not so much subject to infectious diseases. In the hospital, in spite of very poor sanitary conditions, there was hardly a real epidemic, and those that occurred were milder every year. At the beginning of 1940 we had an epidemic of chicken pox in the hospital that lasted 6 months. Almost all the children were affected. At the end of 1941 there was one case and only two children out of 250 caught it. The children in that group were older than those in 1940, but they were terribly undernourished. In other institutions where the food situation was better than at our hospital the percentage of chicken pox infection was as high as under normal conditions. As for scarlet fever, it is a well established fact that well fed children catch the disease more readily. Our children rarely had scarlet fever. The only time we had a number of cases in our hospital was when refugees from Germany arrived who were much better nourished than our children. Measles was also connected with a sporadic influx of refugees to Warsaw. It was rare in the ghetto, obviously because there was such a small increase in population. Meningitis was on the increase at the beginning of 1940, but was very rare after that. The course of the infectious diseases was less symptomatic because of the low reactivity of the organism. Fever was generally low and skin eruptions meager, but the child grew sicker and died. In spite of the lack of usual symptoms, infectious diseases were for malnourished children just a nail in the coffin.

There were few allergic reactions like rheumatic fever, bronchial asthma, or serum sickness. Before the war, during late winter and early spring, a large percentage of our patients suffered from rheumatic fever. During three years of war we saw only five cases, two of which were just exacerbations of previously acquired symptoms.

The course and prognosis in hunger disease are conditioned by many factors, such as the duration and intensity of hunger and the constitution of the child. The younger the child, the more severe the disease. The mortality among infants was almost 100%. Malnutrition with edema had a worse prognosis than dry hunger (cachexia). Edema in five to six year old children was usually a sign of permanent damage and often resulted in death.

EDITORS' COMMENTS

Myron Winick, M.D.

In 1934, five years before these investigators began making their observations, Cicely Williams reported her now classic findings describing a form of protein-calorie malnutrition in children characterized by edema, skin lesions, lightening of the hair, growth failure, and hypoproteinemia. She named this disease kwashiorkor (African for disease of the displaced child) because she noted that it characteristically appeared at the time an infant was displaced from the breast by the appearance of a new infant into the family. She demonstrated convincingly that this disease was caused by protein-calorie malnutrition and not by any specific deficiency in a vitamin as had been postulated by others. Thus, by the time the investigations reported in this chapter were undertaken, two types of severe undernutrition were already known in young children—marasmus, the dry form in which muscle wasting, growth failure, and progressive emaciation predominated, and kwashiorkor, the "wet" form, in which marked edema was the most noticeable sign.

It is not known whether these investigators knew of Williams's observations. However, what they describe in the edematous type of hunger disease in children certainly can be viewed as a variant of kwashiorkor. The authors point out that this form of hunger disease was rare before the age of two and after the age of five. This conforms exactly to the peak age incidence of kwashiorkor in almost all countries where it has been reported. The children were subsisting on 800 calories per day and the diet was extremely

low in protein, which was almost entirely of vegetable origin. This is the
typical low protein, low calorie, relatively high carbohydrate diet that pre-
cedes kwashiorkor. Growth failure was profound, again a cardinal sign of
kwashiorkor, and the children appeared less emaciated than they actually
were because of the edema. The skin lesions that are described are consistent with kwashiorkor, but the flaking and desquamation and the fact
that they appeared as well in the dry form of hunger disease suggest the
possibility of another etiology. The very low fat content of the diet could
have led to a deficiency in essential fatty acids, which could have mani-
fested itself in this type of skin lesions. One difference from the classical
variety of kwashiorkor was the presence of peritoneal and pleural effusions.
Until recently it was felt that the presence of these effusions indicated a
complication and was not part of the primary disease. However, in a study
of Egyptian children it was clearly shown that protein-calorie malnutrition
alone could cause profound ascites in children as part of a picture of generalized edema and that the ascites would disappear with proper feeding.
This observation was made by the physicians in the Warsaw ghetto almost
thirty years earlier. They point out that the differential diagnosis between
these effusions and effusions due to secondary disease was often difficult.
This was particularly true in the case of tuberculosis. However, from their
clinical observations, pleural and peritoneal taps, and autopsy data, they
were certain that most of their children developed these effusions as part of
their primary disease—the edematous form of hunger disease. This observation suggests something which has been recently postulated—that kwashiorkor in infants and hunger edema in adults may form two extremes on a
spectrum and that many older children subjected to severe protein-calorie
malnutrition may show manifestations of both syndromes.

    The study, of necessity, was almost entirely clinical. Even the few in-
struments available for the studies on adults were not available to the workers in the Children's Hospital. Hence, no extensive attempt could be made
to ascertain the cause of the edema. The authors suggest that the hypervolemia described in the adult patients was also present in their children.
They point out that the skin-water test (Aldrich-McClure) was distinctly
abnormal, especially in the edematous children, with the blister disappear-
ing in less than half the time that it does in normal children. Presumably
the extracellular space was enlarged. Today we know from direct measurements that this is true. Another finding that they describe is the severe
limitation in concentrating ability of the kidney. This too has been quan-

titated today but the exact etiology of this concentrating defect is still not completely understood.

Most of the patients described had the dry form of malnutrition, what we refer to today as marasmus. The description by these investigators is extremely detailed and their observations could readily provide a textbook picture of the disease. They note that all of these children fail to grow but that their emaciation and reduced weight far exceeds their retardation in height. Thus the weight : height ratio is reduced, a cardinal finding in severe marasmus. Moreover they note the marked reduction in skinfold thickness and the persistence of that reduction. This was before calipers were used and in fact before skinfold measurements were being made for quantitating changes in marasmus. They also note the lack of subcutaneous tissue and the atrophy of muscle, leading to extreme thinning of the arms and legs. Again this was almost 20 years before Jelliffe introduced the midarm circumference measurement as a way to quantitate protein-calorie malnutrition. They note skin changes that have not been universally noted in children with marasmus. These include vascular changes leading to cold cyanotic extremities, as well as changes in the character of the skin, which was dry, flaky, and desquamating. This could have been a manifestation of essential fatty acid deficiency, which had not been described at that time. They noted dark pigmentation around old scars and on the back and belly. This is certainly not characteristic of marasmus as seen today and I am not sure what it might be ascribed to. They note increased hair growth around the neck and on the cheeks, another observation that is not characteristic of the marasmus seen in developing countries today.

They note the prominence of the lymph glands in many areas and ascribe this to the frequency of skin infections. From the evidence that they present I would speculate that because of the crowding and poor hygienic conditions, skin infections were almost a universal finding and that some of the changes they describe in both the skin and the superficial lymph nodes were secondary to infection rather than a primary nutritional disorder.

In terminal cases enlarged parotid and submaxillary glands were noted. They were not tender and no sign of inflammation was seen around Stenson's ducts. Whether this was true hypertrophy of the gland, silent inflammation, or simply a relative enlargement due to the emaciation and atrophy of the facial muscles is unclear. However, this relative sparing of the salivary glands has to my knowledge not been previously described.

The general wasting of the musculature is a well known finding in this syndrome but the contractures described both in the children and in the adults are certainly not usual in marasmic children. Subsequent to the observations made in the Warsaw ghetto, these contractures were described in concentration camp victims and are discussed in the detailed studies made by the Danish physicians of prisoners returning from several concentration camps. The physicians in the Children's Hospital in the Warsaw ghetto note that contractures appeared only after prolonged semistarvation, which may explain their absence in subsequent controlled human observations in volunteers, such as the Minnesota study by Keys et al. They postulate that the atrophy of the flexor muscles was greater than that of the extensor muscles and that prolonged inactivity in the fetal position allowed the actual contractures to take place. They also postulate biochemical changes in the muscles themselves, but do not speculate any further. Thirty-five years later a host of biochemical changes in muscle have been described and today this constitutes one of the most active areas of research in malnutrition.

The bones are described as both clinically and radiographically normal. This is hard to believe in view of the profound growth failure. I would assume that bone age was not compared to chronological age and that had this been done retarded bone age would have been noted. Unfortunately none of the actual X-rays could be included, so that this important radiological finding must remain obscure. Some evidence of decalcification is described in a few children and this is not surprising in view of the very low level of calcium in their diets. What surprised the authors was the lack of any clinical or radiographic signs of rickets. They point out that this finding was different from the experience during World War I, when rickets was rampant. They ascribe the absence to the immediate administration of vitamin D to children seen in the clinic or admitted to the hospital. An alternative explanation, which is perhaps more likely, is that the degree of malnutrition was so severe that growth ceased almost entirely in these children. Rachitic changes are most pronounced when growth is normal and vitamin D is absent. In addition many of these children were poorly clothed and spent considerable time outdoors (often foraging for food). This exposure to sunlight would also protect against rickets. Whatever the reason for the absence of rachitic changes, similar findings have subsequently been described from all over the world. Rickets is not a usual finding in severe protein-calorie malnutrition in children. The absence of scurvy both clinically and radiographically is also noted. Again this finding is consistent with what has been reported from developing countries. Presumably the metabolic adaptations that occur in the body during semistarvation reduce the need for ascorbic acid. A final observation on the lack of specific vitamin deficiencies was the absence of the characteristic eye and skin changes seen in vitamin A deficiency. This is discussed in much more detail in Chapter 6, although the possible reasons are not discussed. One might assume that since these children, especially the older ones, were reasonably well nourished before the war (unlike most children in developing countries) they had built up significant reserves of vitamin A prior to contracting hunger disease. In addition the vegetable content of the diet may have been significantly higher than that in certain areas where vitamin A deficiency is common and β carotene may have been available. Finally, vitamin A requirements, like those for other vitamins, might decrease during semistarvation. Vitamin A deficiency is still a serious problem today. Many children in Asia with protein-calorie malnutrition show clear signs of vitamin A deficiency. By contrast, most children with protein-calorie malnutrition in Africa do not. The difference presumably is in the availability of small amounts of vitamin A or β carotene in the diet. The children in the Warsaw ghetto resembled the African children in this respect.

The symptoms in the respiratory system are described as shallow regular breathing, lowering of the lung borders, a decrease in breath sounds, and general emphysema. In some children attacks of dyspnea similar to asthma also occurred. These symptoms usually occur only as a terminal event in marasmus and though it is not stated, I assume that these findings were present only after a long period of hunger disease.

The circulatory system showed changes similar to those described for adults. Bradycardia and hypotension were common. Cyanosis, cold extremities, and collapsed veins were present. These findings have since been confirmed in adults by direct measurements of venous and arterial pressures. The pulse pressure often was decreased (another finding subsequently confirmed), and this decrease was regarded as a bad prognostic sign. The authors also describe extra systoles and other types of arrhythmias and regret their inability to perform electrocardiography. The kinds of arrhythmias described are consistent with potassium deficiency, now known to occur in children such as these, especially those suffering from diarrhea. Atrophy of cardiac muscle occurs in both adults and children with severe semistarvation and could also lead to irregularities in heartbeat.

The authors describe a hypochromic microcytic anemia of moderate degree and comment that the degree of anemia must be modified because of the "dilution" of blood secondary to hypervolemia. The white blood cell count was low normal and shifted to the right. The observation is made that eosinophilia was essentially absent, even in children with severe parasitosis. This finding has subsequently been confirmed in developing countries where both malnutrition and parasitic infestation are common. To my knowledge, this is the first time the lack of eosinophilic response has been carefully documented. Platelet counts, bleeding time, and capillary fragility were all found to be normal in these children.

The diarrhea that accompanied hunger disease in children was an almost universal finding. The authors, with limited bacteriological facilities, could not examine all stools, but in those that were looked at, enteric pathogens were not often found. They conclude that the diarrhea in many cases was part of the primary disease and not secondary to infection. This important observation has been confirmed in a number of studies throughout the world. Although cultures must be taken to exclude enteric infections, they are often negative and the diarrhea responds to sound nutritional therapy.

Examination of the nervous system revealed marked psychological changes in the children. They were extremely apathetic and often appeared retarded in their development during the acute early phase of hunger disease. Later these symptoms reappeared as the terminal phase of the disease approached. The investigators conclude that no permanent damage could be demonstrated. We have come a long way since those observations. We know that cellular changes can be induced in the brain if the malnutrition is severe enough and if it occurs during the first two years of life. The patients in this investigation were older. In older children and even in the younger ones we cannot demonstrate that undernutrition per se will result in permanent brain damage. Certainly as part of the complex of poor environment seen in developing countries it contributes to later behavioral abnormalities. However, in better socioeconomic environments it has been shown that even if malnourished early in life, these children recover almost completely. What the results of the ghetto experience on these children would have been we probably never will know. Few survived. Those who did may be scattered all over the world and may have been subjected to varying subsequent environments. Certainly the general impression gained from observations of survivors has been that although certain psychological scars may have been left from the experience, mental development has been normal.

Galvanic stimulation showed decreased motor neuron excitability in 10 children tested. This finding has been reported subsequently in a number of studies, but again to my knowledge this report is the first.

A lack of physiological response to both adrenalin and pilocarpine, coupled with the bradycardia, low blood pressure, and respiratory arrhythmias, suggested to the authors that the autonomic nervous system was refractory to excitatory stimuli and that the vagal system was more affected than other parts of the autonomic nervous system. This observation has been subsequently reported in adults both by the Danish workers and by Keys et al.

The reported delay in sexual maturation and the lack of menstruation in adolescent girls confirmed previous observations and has been reaffirmed many times since.

One of the most important observations made by these workers concerned the interaction of hunger disease and infection. They point out that tuberculosis in all forms was particularly common in these children. The disease progressed very rapidly, causing decompensation rather than the typical adult chronic form of the disease. The authors note that epidemics of measles and chicken pox were rare, a surprising finding unless one assumes that the survivors were already immune. Possible immunity is suggested by the fact that influxes of new people did bring such epidemics with them. When these diseases did strike, they evoked few symptoms. Fever was hardly elevated, rash was minimal, and yet almost invariably the child died.

Two observations made by these investigators have turned out to be extremely important and perhaps had they been known, would have launched the extensive research into the relation between malnutrition and the immune response much earlier. Tuberculin tests were negative even in children with known tuberculosis. Other skin tests (the precise ones are not stated) were also negative. The authors postulate that the typical anergic response was in some way blocked in these patients. Today we know that cellular immunity, which controls these skin reactions, is markedly impaired in malnourished children. In addition, the observation that the lymphoid glands, especially the tonsils, were atrophied agrees very well with this reduced cellular immunity. The second important observation was that allergic diseases such as asthma, rheumatic fever, and serum sickness occurred very rarely. This may be another manifestation of the lack of immune response or it might have been due to the high levels of corticosteroids in patients with hunger disease (not discovered until later) and the suppression of these allergic diseases by corticosteroids, which today has become the standard mode of therapy.

Thus in their short entirely clinical report on hunger disease in children, these investigators meticulously report what they saw and what they could study with the limited equipment at their disposal. They not only give a graphic description of hunger disease as it occurred in the Warsaw ghetto but they make a number of observations which were new at that time. Some of these observations, if previously available, no doubt would have suggested lines of investigation sooner than they occurred. One can only look in awe at these dedicated pediatricians and wonder what they would have learned had they had the time and equipment necessary for the proper treatment of their patients.

Michael Katz, M.D.

This book can be read on two levels, as a scientific treatise and as a document of heroic human endeavor. It qualifies as a remarkable work on both counts. The truism that technology is not the essence of science finds yet another affirmation in this book. One is struck, reading it, by the clarity of thought, by the rational, critical analysis of the observations, and by the persistence and tenacity of the observers. Not given to depression, apathy, or self pity, these investigators struggled to the end and when they were no more, their labor remained and their wish—their prophecy—"Non omnis moriar" has been amply fulfilled. They, our colleagues, have earned immortality.

I have been asked to comment about the observations relating to host defense among the malnourished. This subject has received much attention during the past two decades and we now know a good deal about the handling of infection by the malnourished organism, and about the influence of infection on the nutritional status. The information available today derives both from the development of clear concepts of immunology and from the understanding of metabolism. The recent nutritional and other health related programs in the developing countries have been the impetus for investigators of the infection-malnutrition complex and have thus provided the necessary foundation for the studies of host defense and malnutrition.

Our current knowledge is still incomplete, but many basic facts have been established. It is clear that the cell-mediated immune response is the defense mechanism most affected by malnutrition. Only in extreme cases and in the premortal state can failure of humoral immunity be demonstrated. Thus the malnourished tend to have a reasonably good response to artificial immunization, but what remains unresolved is whether they are subject to any unusual long term consequences of infection with the attenuated vaccine viruses, because their cell-mediated response is blunted.

Within the T cell system there is impairment of function, reduction in the quantity of lymph tissues, and probably a reduction in the absolute number of T lymphocytes. This has its expression in relatively poor reactivity to BCG vaccine and in decreased transformation to blast cells and consequent decreased incorporation of thymidine into DNA in the presence of mitogens. Interferon synthesis has also been deficient in artificially malnourished experimental animals. Both the phagocytic system and the complement system have been shown to be deficient in the states of malnutrition, but these observations require confirmation. Indeed the variability of results deriving from various studies suggests that the malnourished populations were not equivalent and that some host defense functions fail in certain states of malnutrition—perhaps after a certain level of malnutrition has been established—but not in others.

The major unresolved question regarding the relationship between malnutrition and infection is what immune failure can be traced to deficiency or absence of *specific* nutrients. In all of the studies currently available malnutrition has been viewed in its totality. Until more specific and experimental studies are carried out, we shall remain uncertain about the most intimate mechanisms of malnutrition that lead to specific immune failures.

In 1942, the state of relevant biomedical knowledge was primitive by comparison with what we know now. Yet several of the observations reported in this book match those made "anew" two decades later.

Perhaps the most dramatic of these findings was observation of anergy to tuberculin protein, which the authors document and use to explain the fulminant nature of clinical tuberculosis and its high prevalence in the population they studied. Although at the time they did not understand the specific mechanisms of delayed hypersensitivity, the investigators were not satisfied with the mere observation. They considered the possibility that the reaction did take place, but that the skin reactivity was reduced, although not entirely abolished, but because conjunctival response to tuberculin protein was also absent, failure of the host's reactivity to the tuberculin had to be systemic. The issue was not to surface again until the decade 1965 through 1974, when modern technology and current background knowledge resolved the puzzle and showed that failure to respond to the tuberculin protein was a characteristic of the severely malnourished and that it was not the result of failure of skin reactivity.

Not content with this single set of observations, the Warsaw investigators noted that the malnourished had "spontaneous recovery" from various allergies, which was in accord with the postulated failure of immune mechanisms. This exploration of other possible expressions of a phenomenon observed exemplifies the elegance of analytical thought that characterized these scientists.

Other observations of failure to mobilize polymorphonuclear cells, absence of eosinophilia in parasitic infections, the high prevalence of pyogenic infections, the frequency and severity of skin infections, have all been made among the malnourished in the developing countries, some before World War II but most subsequent to it.

This book, containing so much information that we associate with recent literature, has of course some formulations that cannot be supported by our current knowledge. For example, the authors' speculation about the role of the thymus gland must be viewed from the historical perspective of the 1930s. These old points of view are interesting in their own right, but it would be a major error to consider this book an historic relic. It contains much information still useful today, either directly or through its heuristic value. The historic worth of the book centers on its attestation to the wonder and resilience of the human spirit.

THREE Metabolic Changes in Hunger Disease

Dr. Julian Fliederbaum

with the collaboration of

Dr. Ari Heller
Dr. Kazimierz Zweibaum
Suzanne Szejnfinkel
Dr. Regina Elbinger
Fajga Ferszt

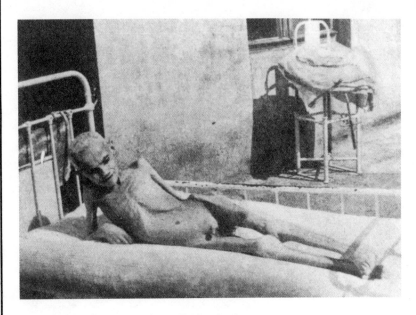

Dry cachexia.

As we have stated before, hunger results in both functional and anatomical changes. These changes result from a lack of necessary nutrients and proceed to irreversible tissue and cellular damage.

Since metabolic studies of hunger disease patients might explain the origins of some of the changes, such studies became one of our central interests. The studies that we conducted are summarized below.

CARBOHYDRATE METABOLISM

Determinations were made on 20 adult and 20 pediatric patients. Since there were no quantitative differences between the groups, we pooled all the data. To interpret the quantitative differences adequately we would have to have studied at least 100 people. We concentrated on carbohydrate metabolism, since many studies during World War I were done on proteins and lipids. Those studies indicated that oncotic pressure was low. In addition protein and lipid determinations sometimes revealed elevations in the level of cholesterol. We found a decrease in total serum proteins (measured with the Pulfrich spectrophotometer). During the research conducted in 1941 we found a low concentration of total protein, a normal concentration of globulin, and a very low concentration of albumin.

Our studies on carbohydrate metabolism included the following determinations:

1. Levels of glucose in capillary and venous blood both in a fasting state and after a 50 g glucose load (smaller load in children) (Figure 1).
2. Glucose tolerance curve in venous and capillary blood after a subcutaneous injection of adrenalin or insulin.
3. Localization of glucose in venous blood.
4. Glucose tolerance after an oral sugar load.

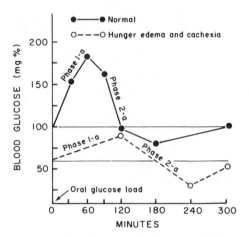

Figure 1   Glucose tolerance test in normal individuals and in patients with hunger disease.

5. Respiratory quotient after administration of an oral sugar load.

We observed many symptoms of hypoglycemia—general weakness, tiredness, reduced physical effort, and somnolence, often accompanied by ravenous hunger. There were cases of spontaneous recovery from diabetes in people on the inadequate diet consumed during the war. By contrast, diabetes persisted in some cases even on a normal diet. All of these observations demonstrate the complexity of carbohydrate metabolism in hunger disease and cachexia.

Glucose tolerance and glycosuria were examined in 20 cases. In normal subjects after a 200 g sugar load, there is usually sugar in the urine (glycosuria). We observed this in only 10% of our patients. Possible reasons for this increased tolerance are listed below.

1. Reduced absorption from the digestive tract perhaps due to an inability to split sucrose into glucose and levulose.
2. Trapping of glucose in the liver and therefore an inability of the glucose to reach the general circulation.

3. Immediate removal of glucose after it reaches the general circulation by starved organs such as the brain, the heart muscle, the liver, the skin, or the striated muscle.
4. Retention of sugar in the blood because of an increased renal "barrier."
5. Rapid oxidation of sugar and hence its utilization before reaching the kidney.

The normal level of pancreatic diastase in urine excludes the possibility that all of the sugar passes through the digestive tract. In addition carbohydrates in food did not stimulate loose bowel movements.

In the present state of science it is difficult to judge whether abnormal sugar absorption from the digestive tract can be connected with disorders in phosphorylation, such as lack of aneurin or cortin.

RESPIRATORY QUOTIENT

Respiratory quotient (RQ) in hunger disease was examined in 70 cases. It is usually high (0.90 to almost 1.0). The reduced excretion of nitrogen in the urine and the RQ near 1.0 strongly suggest that carbohydrate exclusively is being burned in hunger disease. The organism has already burned all its fat and has not yet started to use its own proteins. Within 2 hours after a 100 g or 200 g sucrose load there was an increase in protein free RQ from 0.85 to 0.95, demonstrating that within these 2 hours sucrose was not only split and absorbed into the circulating blood but was also promptly burned (Figure 2).

Basal metabolic rate was measured with the apparatus described by Laulanie-Plantephola. Air samples were taken from glass vessels connected to the gas meter which measured lung ventilation. Normally RQ is 0.85 ± 0.05. Low RQs (below 0.70) are found in the final stages of a short fast or in diabetic acidosis. High RQs, excluding technical errors, appear during enhanced burning of carbohydrate after injection of adrenalin

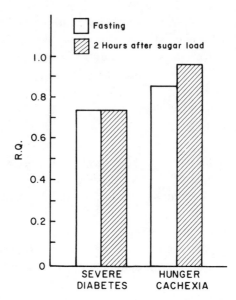

Figure 2 Respiratory quotients in severe diabetes and in hunger cachexia.

(Luska and Riche) and after an oral carbohydrate load in normal individuals where, according to Harris and Benedict, there is an increase from 0.83 to 0.85.

In severe diabetes after an oral carbohydrate load RQ does not increase, demonstrating a loss in the ability to burn carbohydrate (Benedict and Joslin) (Figure 2). In severe diabetes treated with insulin RQ increases from 0.74 to 0.90, which demonstrates the enhanced burning of carbohydrate as a direct effect of insulin (Banting, Best, Collip).

BLOOD SUGAR LEVELS

We measured duplicates of about 85 samples of venous and capillary blood from adults and children. The level of fasting sugar is usually lower than normal (the lower limit of normal is about 80 mg %). In most of our cases levels below 60 mg %

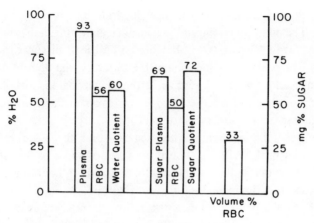

Figure 3   Percent sugar and water in plasma and red blood cells in patients with hunger disease.

and sometimes from capillary blood as low as 32 mg % were seen.

In hunger cachexia and hunger edema symptoms of hypoglycemia often appear spontaneously. This is in accord with the modern concept that hypoglycemia stimulates the sensation of hunger. However, even in severe hypoglycemia from other causes, such as in insulinomas, the level of blood sugar rarely drops so low. These low values are not the result of secondary changes, such as the dilution of blood, because even desiccated red blood cells have low values (Figure 3). Glucose level in adult blood was determined according to the method of Hagedorn and Jensen and in children's blood according to the method of Bang. Free flowing venous blood, as well as fingertip blood was used. Normal levels of fingertip blood range from 80 mg % to 120 mg %. Lower levels are not accepted by many researchers.

GLUCOSE TOLERANCE

We examined 45 samples of fingertip blood after a 50 g oral sugar load (less for children) serially for 5 hours. This method allows for a thorough study of carbohydrate metabolism in humans. The first, ascending, phase in normal fasting individuals reaches 80 to 100 mg %. Following an oral load of sugar, and with the help of the frontal lobe of the pituitary, the thyroid, the adrenals, and the neural centers in the diencephalon, carbohydrates are released from the glycogen reservoir in the liver. This is to counteract the effect of insulin.

The second, descending, phase starts after the sugar level reaches its peak. Within 2 hours the level of sugar in fingertip blood drops below the fasting level and within 3 hours the decline continues if pancreatic function is normal.

This second phase expresses the action of endogenous insulin excreted by the pancreas into the circulating blood, due to the high level of sugar in the blood. It includes the glyconeogenic effect of insulin, which causes storing of glycogen in the liver. In diabetes the second phase of the curve is rather flat with no level of sugar dropping as low as the fasting sample. The descending portion of the curve differentiates diabetes of pancreatic origin from renal diabetes.

In hunger disease besides the low fasting blood sugar levels the curves after an oral glucose load are flat and slow. The peak is reached in about 1.5 to 2 hours, and the descent is very slow. In 3 to 4 hours the level drops below the fasting level to 20 to

TABLE 1   GLUCOSE LEVELS OF A
40 YEAR OLD MAN AFTER A 50 G
GLUCOSE LOAD, SHOWING
OBVIOUS HYPOGLYCEMIA

Time	Blood Sugar (mg %)
Fasting	50
30 minutes after glucose	65
60 minutes after glucose	72
90 minutes after glucose	78
120 minutes after glucose	88
180 minutes after glucose	65
240 minutes after glucose	30(!)
300 minutes after glucose	40

25 mg % with concomitant symptoms of hypoglycemia (see Figure 1). For example, a 40 year old male after a 50 g glucose load had the levels shown in Table 1.

In order to extend our study (Figure 4) we examined the effect of adrenalin on the first phase of the glucose tolerance curve. To study the second phase, we applied the Radoslaw method, which consists of injecting 14 units of insulin and then measuring blood glucose (Figure 5).

In 10 cases 1 adrenalin ampule (Parke-Davis) was injected and glucose level in fingertip blood was measured (Figure 4). The curves were flat and slow. A 32 year old female with advanced hunger edema had the levels shown in Table 2.

Ten cases were examined after injection of 14 units of insulin (Iletyn-Roche). The effect was prompt, showing above normal activity without the usual early ascent. It is a known fact that 15 minutes after an insulin injection in normal people there is a

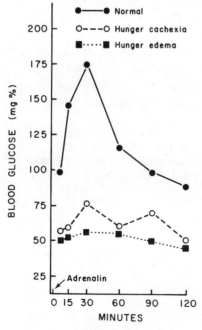

Figure 4   Adrenalin tolerance test.

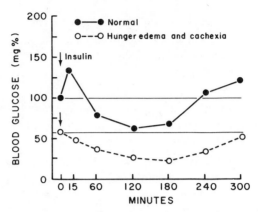

Figure 5   Insulin tolerance test.

fleeting hyperglycemia, secondary to hepatic release of glycogen into the circulating blood. Afterwards the blood sugar keeps decreasing (Figure 5). If the liver is malfunctioning or depleted of glycogen there is no period of sudden increase. In diabetes of pancreatic, thyroid, or pituitary origin, there is no decrease in the sugar level. Figure 5 represents the study of a female patient, 30 years old, with severe edema. The actual blood sugar levels are shown numerically in Table 3.

In hunger disease the first phase of hyperglycemia is flat, showing a slow ascending limb with a flat peak and a flat lazy

TABLE 2   GLUCOSE LEVELS OF
A 32 YEAR OLD FEMALE WITH
ADVANCED HUNGER EDEMA
AFTER INJECTION OF 1
ADRENALIN AMPULE

Time	Blood Sugar (mg %)
Fasting	54
15 minutes after injection	61
30 minutes after injection	75
60 minutes after injection	60
90 minutes after injection	70
120 minutes after injection	48

Hunger Disease

TABLE 3   GLUCOSE LEVELS OF
A 30 YEAR OLD FEMALE WITH
SEVERE EDEMA AFTER INJECTION
OF 14 UNITS OF INSULIN

Time	Blood Sugar (mg %)
Fasting	62
15 minutes after injection	56
30 minutes after injection	51
60 minutes after injection	42
90 minutes after injection	32
120 minutes after injection	32
180 minutes after injection	31
240 minutes after injection	40
300 minutes after injection	58

curve in response to adrenalin. The shape of this curve may be the result of the inhibition of anti-insulin factors, the stimulation of glycogenesis in the liver after a meal or adrenalin, or perhaps the result of a scarcity of glycogen in the liver. Glycogen depletion would also explain the lack of a fleeting early hyperglycemia. The inhibition of anti-insulin factors also could explain the lack of the usual clinical symptoms of insulin shock, such as tremor, anxiety, general feeling of fear, and rapid heart beat. The normal or hyperactive response to insulin suggests a dysfunction of anti-insulin factors.

The clinical picture of insulin shock or spontaneous hypoglycemic shock in patients with hunger disease is different from insulin shock in normal or diabetic persons. None of the above symptoms occurs. Instead, patients with hunger disease exhibit hunger, sweating, and, in the final phase, convulsions and death. Intraocular pressure remains unchanged. The scanty clinical symptoms in spontaneous or insulin induced hypoglycemia, with blood sugar levels as low as 24 mg %, clearly contraindicate the use of insulin in hunger disease.

We planned a series of glycogen determinations in samples of liver, striated muscles, and skin taken right after death. Unfortunately, for reasons beyond our control, it was impossible to pursue this research. Since liver glycogen is markedly depleted, we wanted to examine another rich source of glycogen, namely, striated muscle. Fasting levels of glucose in both venous and capillary blood were examined in 30 cases. In hunger disease there is usually very little difference between the glucose levels in venous and capillary blood, although sometimes slightly higher levels are seen in capillary blood, but within the limits of the method employed. In seven samples capillary blood levels were 20 to 50 mg % less than venous levels in the same patient. Hence in very sick people with low capillary blood sugar levels, glucose goes through peripheral tissues to venous blood, raising its glucose level. Since cartilage does not contain sugar, it cannot be considered a source of glucose. This leaves skin and striated muscle still to be examined as far as carbohydrate metabolism is concerned.

It is not yet known whether glucose is released from striated muscles into the blood by glycogenolysis. According to Parnas, liver is the only source of glycogen. Neither striated muscle nor any other tissue contains glycogen. Pharmacological agents that stimulate the islands of Langerhans will also produce different levels of glucose in capillary and venous blood.

We examined five patients after injection of adrenalin (Figure 6) and five after injection of insulin (Figure 7). Following these stimuli, blood sugar curves in venous and capillary blood

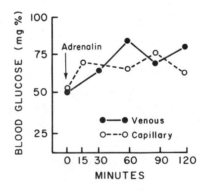

Figure 6   *Venous and capillary blood sugar after injection of adrenalin.*

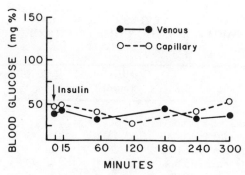

Figure 7 Venous and capillary blood sugar after injection of insulin.

cross each other. In a female 30 years old, fasting levels were obtained after injection of one ampule of adrenalin, as shown in Table 4, and after injection of 14 units of insulin, as shown in Table 5.

We believe that the decrease in glucose levels in capillary blood is associated with a concomitant release of glycogen from striated muscles. Probably glycogen dissociates and forms glucose, which reaches the general circulation through venous blood. We measured glucose levels separately in red blood cells and plasma from venous blood (see Figure 3). We obtained the following results:

1. Percent of red blood cells—33.
2. Sugar in total blood—65 mg %.

TABLE 4   GLUCOSE LEVELS OF A 30 YEAR OLD
FEMALE AFTER INJECTION OF 1 AMPULE OF
ADRENALIN (SEE FIGURE 6)

Time	Capillary Blood (mg %)	Venous Blood (mg %)
Fasting	50	51
15 minutes after injection	70	30
30 minutes after injection	70	65
60 minutes after injection	65	85
90 minutes after injection	75	70
120 minutes after injection	66	81

TABLE 5   GLUCOSE LEVELS OF A 30 YEAR OLD
FEMALE AFTER INJECTION OF 14 UNITS OF
INSULIN

Time	Capillary Blood (mg %)	Venous Blood (mg %)
Fasting	50	41
15 minutes after injection	50	45
60 minutes after injection	42	33
120 minutes after injection	28	40
180 minutes after injection	32	45
240 minutes after injection	43	35
300 minutes after injection	55	40

3. Sugar in plasma—69 mg %.
4. Sugar in red blood cells—50 mg %.
5. Percent distribution of sugar between red blood cells and plasma—72.
6. Water content in plasma—93%.
7. Water content in red blood cells—56%.
8. Percent distribution of water between red blood cells and plasma—60.
9. Water in total blood—81%.

The changes in blood reflect the changes in tissue, since as we demonstrated previously, liver, striated muscle, and other tissues are completely depleted of carbohydrate.

To summarize from our studies of carbohydrate metabolism, we conclude:

1. Glucose in the circulating blood is depleted.
2. Glucose in plasma is higher than in red blood cells.
3. Liver glycogen is probably depleted.
4. There is a diversity of glucose levels in venous and capillary blood with paradoxically high levels in fasting venous blood after administration of adrenalin or insulin. This can be explained by mobilization of glycogen from peripheral stores, for instance from striated muscles.
5. Flat blood glucose curves following a nutritional stimulus

or administration of adrenalin demonstrate depletion of liver glycogen and inhibition of the release or inhibition of the action of anti-insulin factors.

6. Effects of insulin are increased, with blood glucose levels dropping below fasting levels during the descending phase of the glucose tolerance curve. The data demonstrate a normal or even hyperactive pancreatic response.

7. There is an increased tolerance for carbohydrates concomitant with a normal excretion of pancreatic diastase in urine and a normal dissociation and absorption from the digestive tract. This increased tolerance can be explained by:
   a. rapid uptake of ingested carbohydrates by depleted tissues such as blood, liver, and striated muscles
   b. normal or excessive burning of carbohydrates in the periphery.

8. A generally high RQ demonstrates efficient burning of carbohydrates.

9. Respiratory quotient is elevated after the patients are fed cane sugar for 1 week and 2 hours after an oral sugar load.

10. There is a different clinical picture of insulin shock in hunger disease with edema. The alarming symptoms of insulin shock that take place in normal people are absent. Therefore it is dangerous to use insulin for those patients. In addition there is a lack of release or response to anti-insulin factors. Finally, the intraocular hypertension usually observed after injecting insulin does not occur.

We do not believe that such extensive research on carbohydrate metabolism in hunger has ever been previously described in the world literature. Previously published findings were limited to describing low glucose levels in venous blood. For these studies we have employed the most modern laboratory techniques including available micromethods.

Lichwitz detected low blood sugar levels in hunger, an increase after an oral glucose load, and then a slow decrease of the glucose tolerance curve, similar to diabetes. However the clinical material of Lichwitz is utterly different from our patients, who were suffering from endemic, long lasting hunger. Whatever the explanation our observations differ from those of Lichwitz both biochemically and clinically.

We explain the spontaneous recovery from diabetes that occurs during hunger disease as the reverse metabolic response of that which occurs in severely diabetic patients:

1. High carbohydrate tolerance, lack of sugar in the urine even after a 200 g oral load of cane sugar.
2. Low glucose levels in circulating blood.
3. Flat glucose tolerance curve and flat curve after adrenalin injection.
4. Arrest of anti-insulin factors.
5. Distinctive hypoglycemia following a period of hyperglycemia after an oral carbohydrate load.
6. Absence of the usual symptoms of insulin shock with normal or increased insulin release.
7. Normal function of the pancreas.
8. High RQ demonstrating a normal ability to burn endogenous carbohydrate.
9. An even higher RQ after oral ingestion of carbohydrate for 1 week or within 2 hours of an oral carbohydrate load, demonstrating rapid burning of exogenous sugar.

BASAL METABOLIC RATE

Studies of resting metabolism detected some interesting features. It has been known for a long time that during periods of hunger metabolism is lower than in normal individuals and that the effect of proteins is minimal or absent (Labbe and Stevenin, *Metabolism Basale* and L. Lichwitz, *Pathologie der Functionen and Regulationen*).

After carefully examining 70 adults and children we have concluded that resting metabolism was never elevated. In not very advanced cachexia the deviations from normal were within the error of the method (usually around the lower limits of normal—10%). In the second and third levels of cachexia with or without edema, resting metabolism was very low (-30 to -40%), lower than in myxedema. In two terminal patients resting metabolism reached -60%.

These low values are probably due to superficial breathing, decreased lung ventilation, and a low percentage of oxygen consumed. The volume of tidal air per minute in normal individuals is 5 to 6 liters; The percentage of carbon dioxide in expired air is 3 to 3.5%. The percentage of oxygen is 3 to 3.5% and the RQ is 0.80 to 0.90. From this one can readily calculate the volume of carbon dioxide and oxygen in 1 minute or in 1 hour.

In hunger disease the volume of tidal air is 2.5 to 3.5 liters. In the terminal stages it may drop as low as 1.5 liters. The percentage of CO_2 in expired air is 2.4 to 2.6, with a maximum of 2.8 to 3.0. The volume of CO_2 expired in 1 minute or 1 hour was therefore much lower than normal. The percentage of oxygen in expired air was 3.0 to 3.2, rarely as high as 3.4, and the volume per 1 minute or 1 hour was also considerably diminished.

In calculating calories according to Harris and Benedict or according to DuBois the number 700 to 900 points to a considerable lowering of resting metabolism in relation to what is expected.

The observations on RQ (ratio of volume of CO_2 to consumed oxygen) are interesting. In the process of burning carbohydrates ($C_6 H_{12} O_6 + 6 O_2 = 6 CO_2 + 6 H_2O$) the volume of CO_2 equals the volume of oxygen. Therefore RQ (respiratory quotient) is 1.0.

In burning fats more oxygen is used than CO_2 is expired; the RQ is 0.711. For proteins the RQ is somewhere between 0.711 and 1.0. If the RQ is around 1.0, primarily carbohydrate is being burned. If the RQ is around 0.7, primarily fats are being burned. Thus RQ depends on the nature of the organic substance that is being burned during various metabolic processes. Concomitant measurement of urinary nitrogen determines the role of protein and permits us to calculate RQ independent of protein. In order to calculate the number of calories used up by the resting body, an RQ free of protein is essential.

In our patients, RQ varies considerably. In terminal phases of hunger, when body weight loss was 50%, with marked catabolism occurring, the RQ was 0.72 to 0.74. Generally, however, it was much higher (0.95 to 0.98), indicating that carbohydrate almost exclusively was being burned. Three patients were given 300 g of cane sugar daily for a week in addition to their regular hospital diet. The hospital diet was almost the same as their diet prior to admission, about 1100 calories, no fat, low protein (no animal protein). The diet contained mostly vegetables. When these patients were fed cane sugar for a week, the RQ rose considerably. In some cases after an oral load of 100 to 200 g of cane sugar the RQ rose from 0.85 to 0.95 within 2 hours, clearly demonstrating efficient metabolism.

Three patients in addition to their hospital diet received 4 hard boiled eggs daily for a week. Their RQs dropped. A similar drop could be induced within 2 hours of ingestion of 4 to 6 eggs at once.

The data collected on percentage of CO_2 in expired air not only help determine the RQ but also are important in evaluating the acid base balance of the organism. The loss of CO_2 in expired air in 1 minute or 1 hour is much less than in normal people, probably because of reduced pulmonary ventilation and a relatively low CO_2 content in the expired air.

Besides studying the resting basal metabolism we turned our attention to the specific dynamic effects of food. It is known that the thyroid gland is involved in the regulation of basal resting metabolism and that the anterior lobe of the pituitary is involved in regulating the proper dynamic action of food. In normal people metabolic rate increases on the average about 2.8% after eating carbohydrates, whereas after eating proteins the increase averages 26.8%.

Rubner asserts that caloric production by the organism is not dependent on body weight or body surface, but on the quantity of body proteins.

In normal people Benedict and Joslin have found a slight increase after eating carbohydrates or fat and a considerable increase after eating proteins.

According to Manus-Levy, in normal people a protein meal increases caloric production by about 17% of the caloric value of the ingested protein. Our team studied the effects of isodynamic and isocaloric amounts of ingested protein and sugar on 20 adults and 20 children with hunger disease. We did not finish our fat study. In our patients, contrary to what occurs in normal people, within 2 hours of ingesting 200 g of cane sugar, resting basal metabolism increased by 20 to 50%, demonstrating increased burning of carbohydrate. Feeding four to six hard boiled eggs does not affect or sometimes even lowers the basal metabolic rate, demonstrating the lack of a specific dynamic effect of protein in hunger disease. This lack of response could be explained by hypofunction of the anterior lobe of the pituitary or, in some cases, by midbrain vegetative syndromes.

During the war the amount of hyperthyroidism decreased in spite of psychic shocks. This could be related in some way to the prevalence of hunger, which results in a lowering of resting basal metabolism and the abolition of the specific effect of protein, which is increased in hyperthyroidism. We will come back to this interesting subject.

The following findings summarize our studies on the physiology of the quantitative energy changes in hunger disease:

1. Considerable lowering of resting basal metabolism.
2. Lowering or absent specific dynamic action of proteins.
3. Increased metabolism after one or several oral carbohydrate loads. (This finding, combined with the previous finding demonstrating the reversal of the specific dynamic action of food, is especially interesting.)
4. Tendency to high RQ in medium to severe hunger disease and considerable lowering of the RQ in the terminal stages of the disease.
5. Considerable increase in RQ after one or several oral carbohydrate loads, usually occurring within 2 hours after ingestion of sugar; considerable lowering of the RQ after four to six hard boiled eggs daily for a week or within 2 hours of a single load of eggs.

6. Very low minute ventilation in hunger disease, about 2½ liters, even dropping in the terminal stages to 1.5 liters.
7. Lowered amplitude of respirations associated with the low minute ventilation.
8. A slight percentage lowering of oxygen consumption which is partly the result of the low minute volume and partly due to the considerable lowering of oxygen absorption. This conforms to Terroine's law of hypofunction of the circulatory system.
9. Considerable lowering of the percentage of CO_2 in expired air.
10. Considerable lowering of the total amount of CO_2 in expired air, which is due partly to reduced lung ventilation and partly to the reduced percentage.

We shall now discuss mineral metabolism. Even during hunger disease and hunger edema, potassium levels were high and calcium levels low in serum. We had no time to work on cations Na^+, K^+, CA^{++}, Mg^{++}, and their metabolism. We had time to study only the metabolism of chloride, as well as acid base and water balance.

ACID BASE BALANCE

Chloride (Cl^-) metabolism was examined in 20 adults and 20 children. Their food intake was determined according to modern principles. The Cl^- in urine was determined according to the method of Volhardt, the Cl^- in blood and gastric juice according to the method of Rusznyak. The results are as follows: positive Cl^- balance associated with a reduced Cl^- excretion in urine and with a tendency to edema; positive water balance with increased water absorption by the subcutaneous tissue. When food contained 4 to 5 g of Cl^-, 2 to 3 g of Cl^- were excreted in 24 hours. In some patients with normal water balance Cl^- was also normal. In some patients with a tendency to dehydration the excretion of Cl^- in urine reached 7 to 8 g in 24 hours. This demonstrates the well known association between Cl⁻ excretion in urine and the direction of water balance.

It is interesting that as in the edema of cardiac or renal origin, in the edema of hunger disease there is a reduced Cl^- content in gastric juice (30 to 50 mg %). This demonstrates the influence of extrarenal factors, probably of tissue origin, in the etiology of the edema of hunger disease.

In almost all the patients there was a low level of Cl^- in whole blood, 200 mg % (normal 270 to 310 mg %); in plasma, 270 mg % (normal 350 to 380 mg %); and in RBCs, 100 mg % (normal 160 mg % to 210 mg %). The RBC quotient, namely the ratio of Cl^- content in RBCs to plasma Cl^- content, increases, demonstrating that Cl^- migrates from plasma to RBCs.

In summary, the results of our study demonstrate:

1. The well known association between water balance and 24 hour urinary Cl^- excretion.
2. The low Cl^- content in gastric juice.
3. The low Cl^- content in whole blood, plasma, and RBCs.
4. The migration of Cl^- from plasma to RBCs (Zunz-Harburger-Guerber syndrome).

In studying acid base balance we have considered those factors in blood, in urine, in gastric juice, and in expired air which modulate pH. In 20 cases we used the Van Slyke instrument to examine total plasma base. In normal subjects there are 55 to 60 cc of CO_2 in 100 cc of plasma. In hunger disease we did not see any increase above the upper limits of normal. In most cases CO_2 content is reduced, dropping to 40 and even 30% of normal. We did not measure actual blood pH. However, it is known that in severe hunger or prolonged poor nutrition blood pH is low, resulting in acidosis. The abovementioned migration of Cl^- from plasma to RBCs is compatible with our other findings, suggesting an acidosis.

We used the method of Peters and Van Slyke, which measures the quantity of base reabsorbed by the kidneys, to estimate the ability of the individual to eliminate acid. The method consists of titrating a 24 hour sample of urine with phenol as an index and measuring the amount of alkali necessary to bring the pH to 7.4. Since part of the acid excreted is already neutralized by ammonia produced by the kidney, this must be accounted for in the final calculation. The method of Cole was used to titrate the acidity. Under normal conditions, 200 to 400 cc 0.1 N alkali are used to neutralize a 24 hour urine sample. Ammonia in urine was determined by the Folin method. On a meat free diet in a normal 24 hour urine we found 0.170 g. This study was performed on 30 adults and 20 children. At the same time, in 20 cases, urine pH was determined by the Michaels colorimetric method using the Walpole comparator. Urine samples were kept in a cool place and covered with toluene to prevent changes in acidity and the formation of ammonia. The pH of the urine varied from 5.8 to 6.4. Urinary ammonia content was 300 to 500 mg, and sometimes reached 1 g or more. Considering the low caloric diet and carefully calculating the acid and alkaline producing components of the food, we noticed increased amounts of ammonia in 24 hour urine samples. The possibility of technical errors was minimized by reanalyzing particular samples several times. Titrated acidity was very low, 20 to 100 cc of 0.1 N alkali in a 24 hour urine sample.

In hunger disease, especially with edema, reabsorption of base by the kidney was decreased.

In addition to the kidneys the lungs are a very important instrument in removing acidity from the organism through expired CO_2. As we mentioned before, lung ventilation and amount of CO_2 in expired air are always reduced.

Acid loss through the lungs and acid or alkaline loss through the kidneys are stable and irreversible processes. By contrast, the acid secreted into gastric juice is a rapidly reversible phenomenon since within 2 hours of being fed an experimental breakfast patients regularly eliminated alkali into the intestines, momentarily restoring the hydration of the circulating blood to normal.

In 20 adult patients the amount of excreted gastric juice was measured after an alcohol or caffeine load. It is known that in

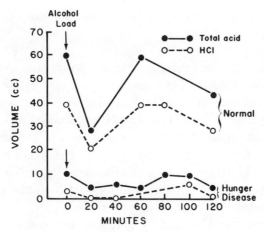

Figure 8   Gastric acidity in normal individuals and in patients with hunger disease.

metabolic acidosis or after physical effort the acidity of the gastric juice increases considerably, whereas in respiratory alkalosis it decreases.

In hunger cachexia, especially with edema, total acidity (A) is low and free HCl (L) was sometimes even absent. Also the volume of gastric juice is much smaller than normal. Figure 8 shows the results of measurements in a 30 year old female with hunger edema. Table 6 gives the numerical values for L/A.

TABLE 6   TOTAL ACIDITY AND FREE HCl IN THE GASTRIC JUICE OF A 30 YEAR OLD FEMALE WITH HUNGER EDEMA AFTER AN ALCOHOL LOAD

Time	Total Acidity/Free HCl
Fasting	2/10
20 minutes after alcohol	0/4
40 minutes after alcohol	0/6
60 minutes after alcohol	1/5
80 minutes after alcohol	4/10
100 minutes after alcohol	6/10
120 minutes after alcohol	4/6

Similar changes were detected in edema originating from causes other than hunger:

1. Low acidity is seen in cardiac or renal edema.
2. Diminished volume of CO_2 per hour is expired by the lungs. There is diminished renal reabsorption of base, resulting in reduced urinary acidity (up to pH 7.4) and normal or enhanced excretion of ammonia by the kidneys (unpublished work by J. Fliederbaum from Prof. W. Orlowski's clinic in Warsaw. In 100 cases of cachexic edema of tumor origin (examined in Vilno) diminished renal reabsorption of base also resulted in reduced acidity of the urine.
3. In cardiac edema there is a lowering of plasma pH as measured with a platinum-hydrogen electrode.
4. Acid base balance is corrected after administration of a diuretic. Specifically, there is an increased retention of base and increased CO_2 excretion and lung ventilation. Gastric acidity increased, renal reabsorption of base was more efficient, and 24 hour titratable acid and urinary ammonia were increased. (Published in a Hungarian paper on mercurial diuresis 1939.)

These data demonstrate a similarity in the disturbances in acid base balance in edema of diverse origin. Is hunger disease characterized by acidosis, or alkalosis? We know that lowered storage of alkali can be the result of respiratory alkalosis or metabolic acidosis. Respiratory alkalosis follows rapid deep breathing and may result in apnea. Expiration of large amounts of CO_2 secondary to deep breathing lowers the CO_2 pressure in the blood, and since the alkali reserve does not change, the pH of blood increases. The organism compensates for this by apnea until the CO_2 pressure returns to normal; at the same time the gastric juice becomes less acid and the alkaline urine contains little or no ammonia.

The ionic equilibrium between plasma and red blood cells is maintained by a diffusion of bicarbonate into the RBCs and a diffusion of an equal number of chloride ions from the RBCs to the plasma. In other words, in respiratory alkalosis Cl^- migrates from RBCs into plasma. Even superficial information present in every handbook is enough to exclude the diagnosis of respiratory alkalosis in our patients—no case history mentions hyperventilation, there was no apnea, ammonia was present in urine, and Cl^- migrates from plasma to RBCs. In metabolic acidosis a diminished alkali reserve could be the result of the flow of endogenous acids into the blood. The disturbed balance expressed by a change in the ratio of H_2CO_3 and $NaHCO_3$ returns to normal, and hyperhydration of the blood stimulates the respiratory center, increasing lung ventilation and reducing CO_2 pressure in the alveolae and in the blood. Under these conditions the pH of blood remains normal because the ratio H_2CO_3 : $NaHCO_3$ remains the same. In our patients we were not able to demonstrate a compensated metabolic acidosis. According to other authors and certain physiological data, severe hunger or long term undernutrition results in acidity of the blood. Indeed in our studies low alkali reserves, migration of Cl^- from plasma into RBCs, and increased excretion of ammonia through kidneys are the signs of metabolic acidosis, but there are some basic differences from the classic form. Our patients do not show symptoms like hyperventilation, which usually occurs in metabolic acidosis as a result of stimulation of the breathing center by acid metabolites. Therefore there is no increased expiration of CO_2 through lung ventilation. In addition, there is no increased excretion of acid through the gastric juice and no increase in 24 hour urine total acidity. Finally, the amount of ammonia is slightly higher than normal, but not as high as in diabetic acidosis, and usually renal reabsorption of base is lowered. The lack of symptoms usually connected with acidosis is probably the result of exhaustion of the organs responsible for the removal of surplus acid from the blood, that is, lungs, kidneys, and digestive tract. This lack of compensatory signs appears to be part of a general insensitivity toward a number of different stimuli; for example, nutrition, changes in body position, physical effort, and adrenalin. Hence the surplus of acids in the blood cannot be excreted because of this general organ insensitivity and, therefore, the metabolic acidosis cannot be balanced.

In order to extend our study we had planned, besides measuring pH of blood, to measure acid metabolites in blood and urine, specifically, lactic acid, ketones, polypeptides, and amino acids. We planned to study the binding ability of protein-lipid complexes from plasma and were prepared to do a complete study of anions and cations. Unfortunately, conditions did not permit us to complete these studies. We can summarize our observations on acid base balance dysfunction as follows:

1. Total base content of blood is reduced (CO_2 usually around 30%). The very low pH in venous blood found by many investigators would indicate a noncompensated metabolic acidosis.
2. An increased amount of ammonia is present in 24 hour urine and Cl^- migrates from plasma to RBCs. These findings also support the diagnosis of metabolic acidosis.
3. However there are no functional compensatory changes characteristic for metabolic acidosis in those organs usually involved in the excretion of surplus acid metabolites. Thus lung ventilation is never increased, expired volume of CO_2 is decreased, and acidity of the gastric juice is very low. These findings are most pronounced in cases of hunger edema. In addition, acidity of the urine reaches pH 7.4 and renal reabsorption of base is decreased. This symptom complex would ordinarily suggest respiratory alkalosis, which has been ruled out by the findings mentioned in items 1 and 2 above.

From these observations we conclude that the metabolic acidosis remains uncompensated because of an insensitivity of certain organs, which is part of the "generalized numbness of the organism." In addition, we would speculate that the uncompensated metabolic acidosis must lead to several types of metabolic derangements.

NITROGEN METABOLISM

Nitrogen metabolism is an important aspect of any study of patients consuming a very low protein diet, especially if their plasma albumin level is low. Some American researchers discovered empirically the effect of sulfur-containing amino acids like cystine, cysteine, and glutathione on hunger edema formation. Unfortunately we did not finish our study. We examined the urine of 20 people, all consuming the same diet containing about 3 g of nitrogen. We measured nonprotein nitrogen (micromethod according to Parnas-Wagner), urea (Hueffner-Ambard), uric acid (Folin-Schaffer Pulfrich spectrophotometer), indican (according to Krebs), ammonia (Folin), amino acids (Folin, spectrophotometer), creatine, and creatinine (Folin, spectrophotometer). Our studies are incomplete because we had no measurements of colloidal nitrogen in urine or in blood, or amino acid levels in blood, and therefore we could not fully examine nitrogen metabolism, but we reached the following conclusions:

1. There is a variable amount of urea. On a mostly vegetarian diet the organism excretes 2.9 g of urea in 24 hours. In our patients, who consumed about 3 g of nitrogen in their diet, urea nitrogen was 2.3 g. In very severe cachexia it rose to 4 to 6 g in 24 hours.
2. There was a reduced amount of uric acid (endogenous) because of a lack of purine nitrogen in the diet. These findings demonstrate diminished degradation of cellular protein. Under normal conditions in a diet devoid of purines the urine contains about 110 mg of nitrogen from uric acid. In our patients it was less than 40 mg.
3. Under normal conditions indican reaches 10 g. In cases without diarrhea the urine contained only half this amount.
4. There was a considerable increase in urinary ammonia accompanying the acidosis and an increased ratio of ammonia to urea, suggesting a role of the liver in these increases.
5. There was an abnormally high amount of nitrogen in urinary

amino acids, sometimes 200 to 300 mg in a 24 hour urine specimen. This can be explained by disintegration of body protein, by a reduced ability of the liver to synthesize protein, or by a decreased ability of the kidneys to produce ammonia (according to the theory that kidneys produce ammonia from amino acids).

6. The reduced quantity of creatinine in the urine is significant. According to Folin, creatinine in the urine of people on a protein free diet is the result of using up the body's own protein. According to Buerger, creatinine index in urine is a measure of muscle work. According to Palmer, Means, and Gamble, there is a relationship between heat produced and excretion of creatinine in the urine. Under normal conditions 600 mg of creatinine are excreted in a 24 hour urine regardless of diet. Our patients excreted 200 to 400 mg in their 24 hour samples, which may be due to the lowered metabolism in the hungry organism. In 17 cases we detected the presence of creatine in urine. Normal adult urine does not contain creatine.

WATER METABOLISM

Water metabolism has not been studied before because of the lack of modern techniques. We used the method developed in Dr. W. Orlowski's clinic, described in many communications in *Polish Arch. for Intern. Medicine* and in *Proceedings of V Congress of Spa Doctors in Krynica, Poland.*

While studying water balance we measured input and output. Input included water contained in solid and liquid food, and that produced by the burning processes in the body. Output included water in urine and feces, and losses through skin and lungs. We also calculated the percent coefficient in water loss from the kidneys and from extrarenal factors. In determining water balance in hunger disease, the volume of circulating water, and the effect of mercurial diuretics on the storage of water in the body, we were able to study the localization of water between the circulating blood and the other body compartments.

The percent of water in the blood was determined from determinations on RBCs and plasma dried to a constant weight, as previously described. We studied the factors regulating the exchange of water between blood and tissues using the method of Hoff and Leuwel (injecting Congo red intravenously and studying the permeability of vessel walls). The ability of subdermal tissue to absorb water was determined according to the method of Aldrich and McClure.

We have already mentioned the increased water content of the blood in connection with changes in protein concentration. Our study was done on 40 adults and 20 children. Water balance varied according to the time of the study. Some patients were in the hospital with edema, and in some, edema increased during their hospital stay. Other patients were completely dehydrated. Regardless of the direction of water balance, the input of water was always increased. The patients were always thirsty, and although the amount of water in solid food and the amount produced as a result of metabolic processes was small, the amount of water consumed as liquid during the day was considerable. The output of water was large as a result of this increased input.

Water loss could be localized as follows: 400 to 700 g were excreted in feces due to the large fecal volume (normal excretion on a mixed diet is 130 g, on a starchy vegetable diet 375 g). Insensible loss through perspiration was normal, 600 to 1000 cc per 24 hours. Excretion of water in urine was markedly increased, reaching 3 to 3.5 liters per 24 hours. The lowest output was 700 to 900 cc. Even patients with edema excreted large volumes of urine, demonstrating the existence of extrarenal factors in the origin of the edema.

The above findings indicate a relative change in the amount of water excreted in the urine. Professor Orlowski's ratio, namely the ratio of water input to water output in urine, was normal. According to Volhardt, after a water load the elimination in urine was normal or even increased. We introduced the ratio of urinary water to the total water loss, which generally increased as a result of efficient or increased excretion of water through the kidneys.

The total amount of intravascular water increases because of the increased amount of circulating blood and the actual percentage of water in the blood. Plasma water increases as a result of the following factors:

1. An increased percentage of water in whole blood to about 94% (normal about 90%).
2. The decreased percentage of red cells in the blood.
3. The relative dehydration of the red cells, which contained 58% water (normal about 65%).

There is an increased amount of extracellular water. Even in clinical examinations the tendency for pleural, peritoneal, and pericardial effusions is obvious. Pricking the skin releases edematous fluid, as occurs when free liquid collects in interstitial spaces, when water is loosely bound by tissues, and in pitting edema. After injection of organic mercurial preparations, for example, salirgan, in patients with hidden or manifest hunger edema, there is a tremendous increase in urinary output in 24 hours accompanied by disappearance of the edema. We believe that mercurial diuretic preparations act upon the stagnant water of the organism.

We mentioned above our measurements of the percentage of water in plasma and RBCs. Since plasma water is increased whereas the red cell is dehydrated, one can assume that water migrates from RBCs to plasma.

The oncotic pressure diminishes because of a lower plasma albumin concentration. Water absorption by the subcutaneous tissue increases. According to Aldrich and McClure, physiological saline injected intradermally takes 60 minutes to be absorbed; in our patients it is absorbed in 10 to 15 minutes. This water absorption is increased even in cachexia without edema. Skin capillary permeability is normal.

In summary:

1. Water balance depends on the clinical condition of the patient. It can be positive, negative, or balanced.

2. Both intake and output of water are increased in hunger disease.
3. The increased input is due to increased thirst and increased intake of liquid food, while the water in solid food and water from metabolism of food is small.
4. The output of water is increased in both edematous and cachexic patients. Renal excretion of water in hunger disease is normal, even in patients with pronounced edema. The ratio of water excreted in urine compared to other routes of water loss demonstrates the importance of the kidney in the process of water loss. In fact, losses through perspiration are normal.
5. Total body water is increased mainly as a result of an increase in plasma volume and stagnation in the Archard cavities system.
6. There is a relative change in water distribution as a result of the migration of water from RBCs into plasma.
7. When discussing the dynamics of water migration from blood to tissues, we must mention the lack of change in the permeability of the capillary walls, the unequal distribution of water throughout the body, and the decreased affinity between water and blood. Water absorption by the subcutaneous tissue increases, and the effects of this are the migration of fluid from the blood to the subcutaneous tissue or into other water reservoirs and the formation of edema.
8. Concomitant with cachexia or hunger edema the following phenomena occur: (*a*) normal diuresis, (*b*) relative increase in the renal elimination of water, (*c*) increased affinity of the subcutaneous tissue for water, (*d*) increase in the quantity of water circulating with plasma, and water stagnating in other parts of the body. In both forms of hunger disease, cachexia as well as hunger edema, both epidermis and mucous membranes are dried out.

The following data are drawn from two patients with hunger disease. Patient B: male, 36 years old, height 169 cm, weight 47 kg (before the war 75 kg), loss 37%. Third degree edema, bilateral pleural effusions, cachexia, and second degree xeransis. On the day of the balance study the diet was composed of 290 g of black bread, 60 g of artificial honey, 15.5 g of sugar, 50 g of rye kasha, 8 g of onion, 8 g of oil, 57 g of oat kasha, 1 g of beans, 24 g of carrots, 71 g of boiled potatoes, 10 g of parsnip, 14 g of cabbage, 5 g of celery, 10.5 g of NaCl, 663 g of water in soup and 600 g in coffee. The weight of the food was 1905 g, protein 44.2 g, fat 16.4 g, carbohydrate 291.6 g, a total of 1525 calories. The water in solid food was 253 cc, in liquid food 1263 cc, from burning food 192 cc, in total 1708 cc. The gain in weight on the day of study was 200 g. Weight of urine was 845 g, of feces 190 g, insensible loss 670 g (skin, lungs). Water eliminated with urine was 796 cc, with feces 149 cc, insensible (skin, lungs) 595 cc. Extrarenal excretion was 149 cc + 595 cc = 744 cc. Input of water was 1708 cc, output was 1540 cc, 24 hour balance was +168 cc. Ratio of water diuresis was 46.2%, elimination of water with urine 51%, extrarenal 49%. Water was absorbed by subcutaneous tissue in 10 minutes. In a 24 hour urine sample there were 9.19 g of urea and 349 mg of ammonia. To reach a pH of 7.4, 83 cc of 0.1 N alkali had to be added.

Patient G: male, 18 years old, height 158 cm, weight 38 kg (before the war 52 kg), loss 27%. First degree edema, second degree cachexia, and xeransis. On the day of the balance study the diet was composed of 22 g of farmer cheese, 54 g of potatoes, 20 g of onions, 50 g of barley, 15 g of beans, 25 g of carrots, 15 g of cabbage, 10 g of parsnip, 4 g of celery, 8 g of oil, 7 g of sugar, 55 g of artificial honey, 2 g of NaCl, 386 g of bread, 545 g of water in soup and 940 g in coffee. The weight of the food was 2168 g, protein 50.9 g, fat 12 g, carbohydrate 312.9 g, calories 1525, Cl 2.74 gm. The water in solid food was 278 cc, in liquid food 1485 cc, from burning food 207 cc. Loss of weight on the day of the study was 1030 g. The weight of urine was 2505 g, of feces 164 g, insensible loss 529 g. Elimination of water with urine was 2422 cc, with feces 129 cc; skin and lung losses were 454 cc. Extrarenal loss was 129 + 454 = 583 cc. Input of water was 1970 cc, output was 3005 cc, 24 hour water balance was −1035 cc. Ratio of water diuresis was 123%, urinary water 80%, extrarenal water 20%. Water absorption into the subcutaneous tissue took 25 minutes. Cl in food was 2.74 g, in urine 10.2 g. Na in food was 8 g. Carbohydrates in food were 313 g, calories 29 per kg body weight. In 24 hour urine there were 6.7 g urea, 843 g ammonia; no alkali was needed to reach pH 7.4.

VITAMIN METABOLISM

Vitamin management was most interesting for us because of its clinical implications. As we mentioned in the first part of this chapter, the vitamin levels in the food were very low and the way in which the food was cooked and stored further reduced these levels. There were disturbances in absorption from the digestive tract in hunger disease because of the lack of HCl in the gastric juice and the rapid passage of food through the intestines. On the other hand, the reduced quantity of vitamins was compensated for by the low caloric diet. We know that the requirement for vitamins is proportional to the caloric intake. We were not able to finish our studies of vitamin balance. Since the food was poor and inadequate the amount of vitamins was also very limited. Even our carefully prepared vitamin balance sheets have no clinical value if they do not coincide with the clinical symptoms of hypo- or hypervitaminosis. Clinical diagnosis of changes in vitamin status requires an exact determination of vitamin balance.

Some of the changes in the skin described above could be due to changes in vitamin metabolism. The dry skin, the tendency to parakeratosis or hyperkeratosis, the diminished immunity of the skin toward infections, the tendency to pyoderma, the changes in nails, hair, sebaceous and sweat glands, the dryness of the mucous membranes of the nose, the poor production of gastric juice, and the arrested growth of the body, are all signs of avitaminosis A. The fact that the diet of our patients was devoid of butter, eggs, milk, and fresh vegetables containing carotene makes this diagnosis even more probable. However, according to Pillat, avitaminosis A does not occur without changes in the eye. These changes appear early and are pathognomonic. Our thorough studies of the eye were completely negative. There was no night blindness, no dryness of the conjunctiva; Bitot spots were absent; there were no changes in color sensitivity. Pillat's spots were not seen in the fundus, nor was there anabrosis of the cornea. Thus the classical symptoms of avitaminosis A were not present.

A lack of vitamin D was also suspected because of the diet consumed. During World War I Warsaw physicians described changes in the bones due to hunger, to a lack of certain food components, and to a lack of light. The changes occurred in tall young men growing rapidly and working hard and in elderly women. The changes in men affected the long bones, whereas the changes in women affected the spine, the pelvis, and the ribs. Compression caused considerable pain in the bony part of ribs, whereas there was no pain in the cartilagenous part. Spontaneous fractures were common. Our hospital patients rarely had spontaneous pain or pressure pain in their bones. The surgeons often saw spontaneous fractures, broken shafts of the femur in young people, poor healing, and poor results when steel pins were inserted because of softening and thinning of the bony tissue. In children X-rays uncovered light areas in the epiphyses of long bones.

We have already mentioned the prevalence of caries in our patients. There were people 20 years old who could not use their jaws because of advanced caries. The most characteristic symptom of vitamin D deficiency, rickets, occurs in children. Our studies did not uncover much rickets in undernourished people during the war. In private practice we saw many cases of painful ribs, spine, and pelvis in elderly women and men, although their diet was adequate but very poor in vitamin D, since they were always indoors. Lack of light is a contributing factor to vitamin D deficiency. Therefore we must conclude that in our experience hunger disease is not usually accompanied by a lack of vitamin D. Dental caries, thinning of bones, light areas in the X-rays of the epiphyses of long bones, spontaneous fractures, and poor healing may be attributed to demineralization secondary to acidosis, hypocalcemia, and hypophosphatemia.

Problems connected with another fat soluble vitamin, E, will be discussed in the section dealing with the sex glands. As far as the water soluble vitamins are concerned, vitamins C and B are best known and have been most thoroughly investigated.

Our patients' diet contained normal amounts of vitamin C. We saw scurvy only once. During the first year of the war scurvy was quite common. This fact can be explained by the theory that to develop symptoms of avitaminosis C a surplus of carbohydrates and adequate calories were important. In typhus and other infectious diseases there were no signs of vitamin C deficiency, though it is well known that those diseases increase vitamin C requirements. We did not see one of the early signs of vitamin C deficiency in our patients, namely, increased permeability of capillary walls.

Vitamin B complex was especially interesting because even a perfunctory study of the patients revealed a number of cases of polyneuritis. Avitaminosis B is suggested by the reduced quantity of vitamin B in the food, but not by the large amount of carbohydrate when compared to amounts of protein and fat. A good diet and large doses of vitamin B_1 helped relieve some of the symptoms of hunger disease. This would tend to confirm the presence of avitaminosis B_1. The B_1 deficiency probably plays a role in the formation of edema in hunger disease. In connection with B_1 deficiency we made the following observations:

1. A wet form of beri-beri (affecting mainly the circulatory system) and a dry form (affecting mainly the nervous system).
2. A sinus bradycardia in hunger disease similar to the bradycardia in avitaminosis B_1.
3. A considerable diuretic effect of intravenous injections of large doses of Betabion [probably a Polish trade name].

In connection with the role of vitamin B_1 in secondary carbohydrate metabolism and in the formation of excess acid and ammonia, we planned to study the excretion of cyclic acids and the levels of pyruvic and lactic acids in urine and blood. Unfortunately we could not do so. It is important to remember that both vitamin B_1 and vitamin C act as diuretic agents in other types of edema, for example, circulatory insufficiency (Bickel). This diuresis is caused by increased absorption of water into the blood, as described previously.

Certain findings in our patients were similar to findings in vitamin B_2 deficiency. Clinical observations in humans have not uncovered pure deficiency of the vitamin B_2 fractions. There are symptoms of lack of lactoflavin, nicotinic acid, or its nicotinamide derivative antipellagra vitamins, vitamin M, and Castle's extrinsic antianemic factor. Those symptoms are *angulus infectiosus oris* (resulting in a burning sensation in the tongue and a smooth base of the tongue), lack of gastric juice, hyperchromic anemia, leukopenia, thrombocytopenia, pellagra-like skin coloring, and acrodermatitis actinica. Not all of these symptoms are observed in our patients. Some, like hyperchromic anemia, are quite rare. Since we have no information on the therapeutic effects of vitamin B_2, we really cannot make any definitive statement regarding the role of vitamin B_2 deficiency in hunger disease.

Summarizing, we can say that in hunger disease there are no signs and symptoms which are pathognomonic for different types of vitamin deficiencies. The most probable deficiency is in vitamin B_1, which may be connected with hunger edema. To our knowledge no therapy with a single vitamin or with a vitamin complex is able to reverse the clinical and biochemical symptoms of hunger disease. These observations are important in view of the small amount of vitamins or provitamins in the food and the possibility of alterations in the absorption of vitamins from the digestive tract in hunger disease. It is possible that with a low calorie diet the need for vitamins in regulating the metabolism of various dietary components is markedly reduced. Antagonism between different vitamins, which is present in a single deficiency, may not occur with multiple vitamin deficiency.

METABOLISM OF HORMONES

The clinical and biochemical changes that occur in hunger disease are sad but dramatic examples of a completely affected organism. There are also many symptoms of impaired endocrine function. Unlike anatomic studies, present clinical methods allow us to measure these impairments. In general, function of those endocrine glands which spare energy is increased whereas the function of those involved in expending energy is decreased. For example the pancreatic islands function well, as does the thymus.

We never observed hyperthyroidism. Graves-Basedow disease was very rare during the war. One would expect that the psychic shock, the conditions of war, and the lack of fat and vitamin A should favor the appearance of Basedow disease, and yet in reality the poor nutrition mostly associated with lack of proteins in the diet prevented hyperthyroidism. Hunger during the war actually produces hypothyroidism. The following are our findings:

1. A marked reduction in energy expenditure accompanied by a low basal metabolism (lower than usually seen in myxedema).
2. Absence of the increase in the specific dynamic effect of protein seen in Basedow disease.
3. Dry, abrasive skin, inclined to parakeratosis (just the opposite of the moist, thin, supple, velvety skin seen in hyperthyroidism).
4. Faint, slow pulse and faint and superficial breathing.
5. Low blood pressure.
6. Increased circulation time.
7. Poor mental level and poor coordination.
8. Flat atrial curve on EKG.

The complex of hypothyroidism is connected with several dysfunctions of basal metabolism after removal of the thyroid gland, described by us, among others, in the Polish literature. The following similarities were observed between hunger disease and hypothyroidism:

1. Low levels of calcium and high levels of potassium in plasma.
2. A tendency to retain water and salt.
3. A reduced water absorbing capacity of the blood due to low levels of albumin.
4. An increased water absorbing capacity of the subcutaneous tissue.
5. An increased carbohydrate tolerance.
6. Low blood sugar levels, flat glucose tolerance curves secondary to nutritional and adrenalin stimulation, and prompt reaction to insulin.
7. Low blood urea nitrogen.

However, not all of the symptoms are identical. For instance, in hypothyroidism the edema is hard and compact. In hunger edema it is doughy, soft, and movable.

There are no signs of hyperfunction of either the adrenal medulla or cortex. Some signs of intersex, as described in Chapter 1, such as lack of distinctive sexual features in adolescents growing up during the war, would also tend to rule out cortical hyperfunction. Our observations suggest that on the contrary, signs of hypofunction are present. The heterosexual hair growth and the presence of hirsutism as lanugo are not always symptoms of abnormal adrenocortical function, since they often occur in tuberculosis and in infantile individuals as part of a multihormonal disturbance.

Analyzing the above symptoms in detail reveals the following similarities with Addison's disease:

1. Psychic asthenia, lack of coordinated thinking, and reduced mental effort.

2. Muscular asthenia, lack of physical strength, desire to stay in bed.
3. Cardiovascular asthenia, drop in arterial, venous, and capillary blood pressure, increased circulation time, and abnormal reaction to changes in position.
4. In addition, atony of the striated muscles, reduced muscle strength, and a tendency to melanoderma, especially after trauma.

There are distinct differences, however, between Addison's disease and hunger disease. For example, there is a different localization of pigmentation in the skin, and whereas the pulse is accelerated in Addison's disease, it is decelerated in hunger disease. In Addison's disease circulating blood volume (mostly plasma volume) is reduced and edema is lacking. In addition, blood urea is usually low in hunger disease, whereas in crisis from adrenal insufficiency it is often elevated. The following similarities can be described in the metabolic changes between experimental hypofunction of the adrenals due to surgical removal of the gland and hunger disease:

1. Low calcium levels and high potassium levels in plasma.
2. Reduced alkali reserve in the blood.
3. Reduced concentration of Cl in total blood and migration of Cl from plasma to red blood cells.
4. Reduced water absorption into blood due mostly to the low levels of albumin in the plasma.
5. Increased carbohydrate tolerance.
6. Low fasting sugar levels and flat glucose tolerance curves after nutritional and adrenalin stimulation.
7. Marked response to insulin; insulin shock without an appropriate adrenal response, which is different from the classical clinical symptoms of insulin shock.
8. Lowering of the resting basal metabolism.

As for the involvement of the parathyroid glands, we often observed caries and striped teeth and trophic changes of the skin and nails, which are symptoms of long lasting hypoparathyroidism. Detailed study often reveals increased sensitivity of the muscles when pinched or struck with a reflex hammer. Chvostek's reflex and low levels of calcium in the plasma were often present, indicating latent tetany or a pretetany state. In children whose acidosis was corrected by injection of salirgan, or in adolescents, mostly during springtime, frank tetany was occasionally observed. This may be due to a sudden decrease in serum calcium and in the acid equivalent accompanied by a decreased volume of circulating water, or to an increased demand for parathyroid hormone, which sometimes occurs in the growing organism. All these factors exhaust already weakly functioning parathyroid glands in hunger disease, and simple hypoparathyroidism changes into tetany. We do not know to what extent a lack of vitamin D may contribute to the tetany, considering the synergism between vitamin D and parathyroid hormone.

In comparing typical tetany with hunger tetany we observed low phosphorus levels, low plasma alkali reserves, acidosis, and an increased volume of circulating blood in hunger tetany. In experimental hypoparathyroidism we also observed increased water absorption due to an increased concentration of albumin in the plasma.

The cataract of hunger disease is different from that seen in hypoparathyroidism. In hunger disease it resembles the cataract of old age and is a symptom of premature aging. Recent results suggest that cataracts are the result of faulty tissue oxidation or tissue acidity.

The function of the sex glands is undoubtedly affected by psychic factors as well as by hunger. During the bombardment of the city and during the days of defeat and collapse, many men become impotent and many women stopped menstruating. In normally fed people these symptoms regress rapidly. In undernourished patients they remain. It is difficult to document vitamin E deficiency in the food, and vitamin A may also be involved, which complicates our understanding of the pathogenesis. In shelters for girls, as indicated by the supervisors, many girls started menstruating upon receiving vitamin A, even if they had not done so for a long time, or even if they had never menstruated because puberty started during the war.

Clinical symptoms may vary in particular cases. Well fed women gain weight promptly when menstruation ceases. Adolescents entering puberty during the war remain generally and sexually infantile. This infantilism is different from the physical and sexual underdevelopment seen in adolescent diabetes. In hunger disease, stunting of growth is equally distributed through the body and the extremities, but the face, unlike that of diabetic children, appears old and can be described as "Gilford's progeria" or "Variot's senilismus." The hair on the face and in the pubic region is heterosexual. There is a lack of hair in boys, a fuzzy moustache and sideburns and underdeveloped pelvic bones in girls. The only remnants of subcutaneous fat are in the pubic symphysis, and there are no changes in the voice. Both sexes are sterile.

In the few cases in which babies were born, the survival rate was very low. In neither sex was a complete castration syndrome witnessed. There was no abnormal growth of the lower extremities, and obviously no fat in the subcutaneous tissue. The pallid, slightly yellow face could also be connected with the inhibition of sexual maturity. In hypofunction of the sex glands, as in our patients, creatine appears in the urine. We did not have time to determine the levels of folliculine and androsterone.

The pituitary gland is also damaged by hunger disease. We are not discussing symptoms connected with the unsatisfactory secretion of hormones which stimulate the thyroid, adrenals, parathyroid, ovaries, and testes. Deficiency of these hormones produces the same symptoms as primary hypofunction of these glands. However, since in hunger disease there is partial hypofunction of the target glands which is different from such classic syndromes as myxedema, Addison's disease, tetany, or castration, the question arose whether the frontal lobe of the pituitary might contain the secret of hunger disease. Could this be Simmond's syndrome or Bickel's disease—benign, easily cured hypopituitarism? Obviously the endocrine disorders of hunger disease are multiglandular. The following specific changes occur in the pituitary Bickel's syndrome:

1. Old, wrinkled face.
2. In some cases a lack of specific dynamic function of protein during very low resting metabolism.
3. Microsplanchia, a shrinking and drying out of organs and tissues, which gives the patients a dwarfish appearance.
4. Hypothermia.
5. Asthenia of the circulatory system.
6. Disorders of metabolism, mainly carbohydrate metabolism.

Arguing against a unique role of the pituitary in hunger disease are symptoms that are better ascribed to malfunction of the posterior lobe and mesencephalon, namely, polyuria in the early stages of the disease and water retention in the later stages. According to research completed just before the war on the effects of biodialyzates of the pituitary frontal lobe, we concluded that polyuria and diabetes insipidus are results of combined hyperfunction of the anterior lobe and hypofunction of the posterior lobe, which regulates the function of the anterior lobe. In the early stages of hunger disease the polyuria results from hypofunction of the posterior lobe, preventing a pituitary diuresis. In the later stages there is also hypofunction of the anterior lobe, resulting in water retention. The facts that the thymus and the pancreas work adequately or even more actively than normal and that the typical skin coloring and edema appear, argue strongly against complete dysfunction of the pituitary. The thymus and the pancreas are organs that protect the body from inefficient metabolism.

The role of the thymus is not yet established, but considering the latest discoveries by Bomskow we can assume that some of the symptoms of hunger disease may be an expression of altered thymic function. Hyperfunction of the thymus is associated with the following findings:

1. Low glycogen content in the liver. Bomskow considers this proof of the existence of a thymus stimulating pituitary hormone.
2. Curbed sexual development of the organism during the growing period.
3. Increased number of lymphocytes in the blood. These are the thymus hormone carriers.
4. A tendency to retain water, as revealed by an increased turgidity of the tissues.

Seyle has described an antagonism between the adrenals and the thymus in that hypofunction of the adrenals is accompanied by hyperfunction of the thymus. It is possible that this is occurring in the growing organism during hunger disease. An essential symptom of thymus hyperfunction, extra growth, has never been noticed in our patients.

The pancreas plays an important role in our research. Besides the obvious alterations in carbohydrate metabolism there is a parasympathetic excess, which may be due to the secretion of vagotonin and to impaired production of sympatonin by the chromafin system. Alterations in carbohydrate metabolism are specific for cachexia and hunger edema. Carbohydrate tolerance is increased. The body takes up sugars rapidly from the digestive tract, promptly absorbs them, and uses them at once, metabolizing them rapidly into available energy. The glycolytic activity of insulin in the hungry organism is more apparent than glycopetic activity. This can be demonstrated if one analyzes the blood sugar curves after insulin injection and in the second or descending phase of nutritional hyperglycemia. There is a low blood sugar level, and a marked lowering of this level after insulin and in the second phase of the curve following an oral glucose load. These findings strongly suggest adequate pancreatic island function.

Our results would also preclude primary hyperfunction of the pancreas, as in insulinomas for example. The secondary hypoglycemia and possible hyperfunction of pancreatic islands is confirmed by symptoms of blunted antagonistic responses, such as hypofunction of the adrenals, the pituitary, and the thyroid glands, and low flat glucose tolerance curves in response to nutritional stimuli and to adrenalin. In addition, the lack of an appropriate response to insulin injection (cardiac palpitations, tremors, an accelerated pulse rate, and the usual psychomotor reaction) also suggests the loss of these antagonistic reactions.

AUTONOMIC NERVOUS SYSTEM

An endocrine profile would be incomplete without a few words about the autonomic nervous system and its connections with centers in the diencephalon, with the endocrine glands, and with peripheral sites. The clinical observations of slightly closed eyelids, withdrawn eyebulbs, narrow pupils, a discrete Claude Bernard-Horner syndrome, slowing down of the respiratory and pulse rate, lowering of the arterial and venous pressure, and relaxation of muscular tonus suggest a paralysis of the adrenergic system.

By contrast, one also observes a lack of cholinergic stimulation to the lacrimal, sweat, and sebaceous glands, as well as to the stomach and biliary tract. However, we cannot rule out the possibility that the lack of function is due to a lack of end organ response in those glands.

As for striated muscles, one observes a narrowing of the pupils of the eye, a lack of tonus in the muscles of the arteries and veins, and increased peristalsis of the intestines. These symptoms are due to a stimulation of the cholinergic system. These findings are consistent with clinical observations suggesting paralysis of the stimulating functions of the adrenergic system and dissociation of the functions of the cholinergic system, resulting in adequate functioning of the striated muscles most concerned with maximum sparing of energy.

Our findings in the field of the autonomic nervous system are:

1. Low tonus of the adrenergic system:
   (a) Absence of pilomotor reflex.
   (b) No "goose pimples" after cooling of the skin.
   (c) Accelerated pulse after pressure on the solar plexus.
   (d) Accelerated pulse and increased pressure (see "swing" test) after physical effort and after hard boiled egg test.
   (e) Lack of red dermography.
2. The response to adrenalin is abnormal:
   (a) No acceleration of breathing or pulse.
   (b) No elevation of blood pressure.
   (c) No increase in blood sugar.
   (d) Absence of leukocytosis.

These symptoms demonstrate not only decreased sympathetic activity but also the inability of the organism to react normally to pharmacological stimulants like adrenalin. In addition intradermal injection of adrenalin did not result in vasoconstriction of the skin. We believe that the feeble reaction to intradermal and intraocular tuberculin, when added to other facts from the literature, also is consistent with a paucity in sympathicostimulating substances.

Examination of the cholinergic system results in the following findings, which demonstrate its low tonus:

1. Pulse is not lowered and blood pressure is not decreased after pressure on the eye (Ashner-Dagnini), massage of the neck branch of the vagus nerve (Tschermak), or the placing of the patient in the Trendelenburg position in our "swing test."
2. Injection of pilocarpine does not induce a normal response such as sweating, salivating, further narrowing of the pupils of the eye, slowing of the pulse, or lowering of the blood pressure.

Hence in hunger disease there is diminished tonus of both antagonistic systems and reduced sensitivity toward vegetative toxins.

A modified Danielopolu test, consisting of injecting atropine into the eye, demonstrates that there is vagotony—an increase in the cholinergic system when there is insufficiency of adrenergic and cholinergic substances—and hypoamphotony in cachexia and hunger edema. The reduced basal metabolism, the diminished calcium level, and the increase in potassium in blood, as well as the low levels of sugar and albumin in blood, support the concept of vagotony.

In previous studies we demonstrated parasympathetic substances in the blood in patients with edema of different origins, diminished water absorption into the blood resulting from vagotonic or sympatheticoparalytic drugs, and an increased water absorbing capacity of the subcutaneous tissue induced by cholinergic drugs.

The results of those studies were confirmed by several authors (Hashimoto, Koichi, Kostyal, and others) and have brought about the concept of a role of the cholinergic nervous system in controlling the retention and elimination of water in the circulation.

The increased parasympathetic activity enhances renal water elimination and also water retention in tissues. In summary, we conclude that in hunger disease there is a prevalence of those factors conserving energy and a reduction of those factors which waste energy.

EDITORS' COMMENTS

Robert Bernstein, M.D. and Myron Winick, M.D.

This chapter is certainly the most sophisticated research undertaking of the entire study. As the author points out, it was the most detailed examination of carbohydrate metabolism ever undertaken in semistarvation and in many ways it remains so. The following measurements were employed during the investigation:

1. Venous and capillary blood glucose after an oral glucose load, after epinephrine injection, and after insulin injection.
2. Respiratory quotient.
3. Basal metabolic rate.
4. Specific dynamic action of proteins.

The techniques and equipment necessary to make these measurements were relatively new in 1940 when this study was done, and when one considers the conditions under which the determinations had to be carried out, the results are truly remarkable.

In addition to investigating carbohydrate metabolism the author investigated acid base balance by examining the metabolism of chloride and the excretion of carbon dioxide. The demonstration of a compensated metabolic acidosis in semistarvation is a careful documentation of what had previously been suspected but never actually proven. The difficulty in carrying out chloride balance studies is hardly even discussed but must have been formidable. Measurements were made in food, plasma, RBCs, urine, and gastric juice. In addition, studies of water balance and measurements of urinary excretion of ammonia were carried out. Even today the collection of such material for research purposes is usually confined to well equipped metabolic wards under the direction of specially trained, highly skilled staff.

Studies of nitrogen metabolism and attempts to carry out nitrogen balance studies were also undertaken. The diet was carefully analyzed on the day of the study and nitrogen was measured in feces, urine, and sweat. The author even attempted "vitamin balance studies," but found that these were not feasible under the prevailing conditions.

We have described in some detail how these studies were organized and the types of determinations that were carried out because the decision to undertake this kind of investigation under the conditions that were prevalent in the ghetto must have been made with full awareness of the odds against getting any really meaningful results. In spite of this, the studies were initiated and carried out meticulously and have given us extraordinary data that have stood the test of time.

These studies were done before any hormone could be measured and before many of the important humoral agents involved in intermediary metabolism were known. By contrast, some putative hormones described by the author, such as thymic hormone, have not been found. Thus the study must rely upon clinical syndromes and secondary metabolic changes. Some of the studies, especially in carbohydrate metabolism, are unique. We will try to interpret them in the light of recent studies in patients with protein-calorie malnutrition or anorexia nervosa, or in normal, usually obese individuals on experimental fasts. None of these conditions entirely replicates this study because dietary composition may vary with ethnic group and location, and superimposed disease may alter metabolic responses. Also, the metabolism of obese individuals differs markedly from that of lean or undernourished patients, and should not be used as a precise model. In particular, there is an abundance of adipose tissue, so that the body is never required to utilize alternative energy sources. Anorexia nervosa is a condition with psychological causes that may alter hypothalamic responsiveness independent of the state of nutrition.

The low levels of fasting blood glucose in the patients in the Warsaw ghetto are similar to those in all studies of semistarvation, and are present despite reduced levels of insulin, normal plasma cortisol, and elevated growth hormone levels. However, specific hypoglycemic symptoms are absent. The author describes weakness, fatigue, somnolence, and hunger, all of which can be ascribed to malnutrition independent of hypoglycemia. He makes no mention of reversal of these symptoms after a sugar load. It is notable that adrenergic symptoms are absent, and neurological sequelae, such as coma or convulsions, are not described.

From the data presented we cannot be certain which body fuels are being used by these patients. The high nonprotein RQ suggests that most of the energy is derived from carbohydrate. Yet a normal man has very limited carbohydrate stores, and must rely on protein or fat for energy not supplied by diet. The reported intake was high in carbohydrate (mostly complex) with little fat or protein, but the ostensible calorie intake was low (estimated at 1100 kcal per day). The reduced BMR probably spares endogenous fuels and allows dietary sources to supply most of the body's requirements. Since the BMR is determined in the postabsorptive state, the carbohydrate that was used must have been supplied by glycogenolysis or gluconeogenesis. The low RQ in the preterminal state indicates depletion of the protein and carbohydrate stores, which had been used up by most of the subjects.

The sugar tolerance may be divided into phases of: (*a*) absorption of sugar; (*b*) utilization, both in insulin-dependent and in insulin-independent tissues; and (*c*) counterregulation, due to the effects of glucagon and catecholamines. The patients with hunger disease demonstrate a flat curve with a late peak, followed by a prolonged fall into a frankly hypoglycemic range (Figure 1). The authors note that the RQ and metabolic rate rise after sugar, and that there is no diarrhea. They correctly infer that the sucrose load is rapidly utilized. The fall to hypoglycemic levels and the slow recovery are ascribed to unimpaired insulin secretion and sensitivity, and to loss of anti-insulin factors. However the response to exogenous insulin (Figure 5) is surprisingly small for a dose of 14 units (approximately 0.25-0.3 units per kg). To our knowledge these are the only data demonstrating the response of patients with prolonged semistarvation to exogenous insulin available in the medical literature.

The endogenous insulin response in total fasting has been well characterized by many authors. It includes absence of first phase release (within 5 minutes of an intravenous glucose load) and delayed or absent second phase release. The result is a diabetic glucose tolerance curve. Grey and Kipnis have shown that as little as 0.5 g glucose intraperitoneally every 8 hours can maintain insulin secretory capacity in a fasted rat, although the

caloric content is insignificant. This may be analogous to the high carbohydrate, hypocaloric diet in the Warsaw ghetto patients. Yet in studies of
protein-calorie malnutrition in South Africa, most patients have had either
no insulin release or subnormal early release with prolonged secretion.
Autopsy data in starved patients sometimes show atrophic islets of Langerhans. However, this was not a consistent finding in this study. Insulin receptors are increased after fasting, and thus sensitivity of some tissues might
be increased; however, the increased sensitivity is not corroborated by the
insulin tolerance data in this chapter. It may be that much of the glucose
is used in insulin-independent pathways. This would explain improvements
in diabetes during semistarvation.

Impaired counterregulation is seen in both sugar tolerance and insulin
tolerance. Although glucagon was unknown at the time of these studies, the
authors accidentally demonstrate the absence of a glucagon response. Thus
the normal rise in blood glucose after "insulin" (Figure 5) is probably due
to contamination with glucagon, since similar findings are not seen with
the purer insulin currently available. This response is absent in starved
patients. The hyperglycemic response to epinephrine is also impaired.
These suggest end-organ failure, probably including glycogen depletion,
and thus the secretory response of these hormones cannot be assessed by
measuring blood glucose. The absence of other adrenergic symptoms after
epinephrine is more suggestive of peripheral unresponsiveness. This might
be due to loss of receptors. The systemic acidosis might also contribute to
hormonal unresponsiveness. However the probable absence of plasma triiodothyronine (T_3), as discussed below, raises the intriguing possibility
that the absent catecholamine response is due to T_3 hypothyroidism. It
would be of interest to compare responses to epinephrine in semistarved
individuals before and after replacement T_3.

The author makes a point of the reversal of the normally positive
capillary-venous gradient of glucose in his patients during insulin or epinephrine tests. He concludes that peripheral tissues must be releasing glucose. Today we realize that this cannot occur, since glucose-6-phosphatase
is present only in liver and kidney. A more reasonable explanation can be
found in the peripheral vasoconstriction found in starvation, which should
be accentuated during epinephrine injection or insulin hypoglycemia. This
will cause: (*a*) shunting of arterial blood away from skin into the venous
effluent; and (*b*) hemoconcentration in the fingertip capillaries with over-
representation of red blood cells in the whole blood glucose. These effects

will combine to make the venous blood glucose levels higher than the capillary blood glucose levels.

The description of acid base balance in this chapter is one of the earliest pictures of the metabolic acidosis of starvation. The authors describe hyperkalemia, hypochloremia, and reduced total CO_2. These are consistent with a high anion gap caused by accumulation of fixed acids (lactate and ketone bodies). The reduction in chloride movement into red blood cells is probably due to the acid base disturbance. However the gastric achlorhydria is more likely due to mucosal atrophy. The low titratable acidity in the urine suggests a degree of renal tubular acidosis, although much of the excreted acid is undoubtedly accounted for by the high ammonium content.

Reduced nitrogen excretion in starvation was not unique to this study, and is an adaptive response of the body. It is known to reflect the preferential use of body fat over protein for energy, with diminished gluconeogenesis. The author describes the typical low urea excretion and high ammonia loss. The former is a result of the reduction in hepatic gluconeogenesis, with glucagon levels reduced to normal postabsorptive levels after an early rise in the first week of starvation. Ammonia excretion reflects renal gluconeogenesis, and is stimulated by acidosis. The low uric acid excretion is partially due to the decreased cell mass and dietary load, but also due to impaired distal renal tubular secretion of uric acid in acidosis.

Impaired calcium metabolism is described in these patients, with radiolucency of bones, spontaneous fractures, hypocalcemia, hypophosphatemia, positive Chvostek sign and occasional tetany. Dietary vitamin D deficiency is certainly present, and lack of sunlight prevents production of this vitamin in subcutaneous tissues. It is not certain whether adipose tissue loss would further impair endogenous vitamin D production. However, the patients show more rapid calcium depletion than could be expected from the dietary deficiency over the duration of the famine. The acidosis may contribute to bone demineralization. As the authors note, correction of the acidosis may cause tetany possibly by allowing remineralization using serum calcium. In addition, these patients may have been deficient in magnesium. This, in turn, could produce impaired parathyroid hormone release and action. Decreased dietary phosphate should cause osteomalacia from reduced mineralization of colloid, but in normal, vitamin D replete individuals there is a compensatory increase in renal production of 1,25-dihydroxy vitamin D. This compensation would not be possible in vitamin D deficiency.

The demonstration of clinical polyneuritis and cardiovascular symptoms

suggestive of thiamine deficiency is also of interest. Thiamine is certainly
needed for utilization of the carbohydrate rich diet. The diuresis after
vitamin injection is good evidence of wet beriberi.

As noted by the authors, starvation produces the clinical characteristics
of panhypopituitarism or of a combined thyroid, adrenal, and gonadal
deficiency. Surprisingly, precise chemical measurements in patients with
protein-calorie malnutrition or anorexia nervosa do not corroborate this
diagnosis. Although such patients show clear-cut evidence of hypothalamic
hypogonadism and subtle thyroid hormone deficiency, the other changes
associated with panhypopituitarism are not present. The thyroid hormone
deficiency has been the subject of intensive recent investigation. In starvation and in chronic diseases, free thyroxine (T_4) levels are normal or only
minimally reduced, but triiodothyronine (T_3) levels are very low. In our
hospital many cachexic patients have unmeasurable plasma T_3. Thyroid
stimulating hormone (TSH) level is normal, and responds appropriately to
thyrotropin releasing hormone. The defect is in peripheral conversion of
T_4 to T_3, and is due to both low calorie and low carbohydrate intake. In
addition, it is quite possible that iodine deficiency would be present in the
patients in Warsaw. The implications of low T_3 are uncertain, since many
tissues respond to T_4 without conversion. However, the low BMR may be
a result of this change. Low T_3 should also decrease the rate of protein
catabolism. This would be consistent with the author's observation that
"in hunger disease there is a prevalence of those factors which conserve
energy." The low T_3 syndrome might be viewed as an important anticata-
bolic adaptation to starvation.

As is evident from our own speculations based on the data reported in
this chapter, a great deal of new information has become available to the
scientific community. Already some of the observations made by the Warsaw investigators have suggested new lines of investigation and no doubt
as the data in this chapter become more widely known, more areas of investigation will be opened. Certain conclusions can be reached from the
study itself. Blood sugar levels in patients with hunger disease are low.
Oral glucose tolerance tests show blunted response with a late peak and a
slow fall to hypoglycemic levels. The usual hyperglycemic response to
exogenously administered epinephrine is not seen and instead there is only
a minimal increase in blood sugar levels. Exogenously administered insulin
results in a much more gradual drop in blood sugar than would be ex-

pected in normal individuals, and the ultimate level of blood sugar that is attained is not as low as might be expected.

From these data it is clear that carbohydrate metabolism is profoundly altered in hunger disease. The data suggest that this change is due at least in part to unresponsiveness of end organs to both epinephrine and insulin. The uncovering of the mechanism by which this adaptive response occurs will undoubtedly provide a challenge to future investigators.

Other clearly documented observations made in this chapter were the low basal metabolic rate and the relatively high RQ in adapted patients, which falls to low levels prior to death. In addition, the normal metabolic response to either a carbohydrate or a protein load is clearly demonstrated. Thus these patients have adapted to their low calorie, relatively high carbohydrate environment but are perfectly able to respond appropriately to exogenous nutrients given either as carbohydrate or as protein.

This metabolic adaptation is further demonstrated in the investigation of the acid base status of these patients. The Warsaw investigators convincingly built a case, based on their own data and on deductions that they drew from the data, for a partially compensated metabolic acidosis in this disease. This has been observed by many investigators since, and actual measurements of acid metabolites in blood have been made, but to our knowledge this was the first extensive series of observations and careful measurements made in this area. At present, we still do not know whether the organism derives any benefit from undergoing this change in acid base balance during prolonged starvation, and as in the area of carbohydrate metabolism, this study raises a number of questions that undoubtedly will be the subject of future research.

The studies of water balance are an attempt to explain the etiology of the edema. Unfortunately the methods necessary to measure total body water and water in the various body compartments were not yet available at the time of this study. Using "indirect" measurements, such as the Aldrich-McClure test, and carefully measuring the total water intake and output, they concluded that water balance was variable. Some patients, especially those with edema, were in markedly positive balance; that is, they retained water. By contrast, other patients, most often those with the dry cachexic form of the disease, were in negative balance; that is, they excreted more than they took in. Thus these investigators were able to demonstrate at least that water balance was extremely variable in this disease. By contrast, the distribution of water appeared to have the same pattern regardless of the type of hunger disease noted. The Aldrich-McClure test demonstrated rapid disappearance of water from a skin blister into the subcutaneous tissues. While the disappearance was somewhat more rapid in patients with the dry cachexic form of hunger disease than in patients with the edematous form, in both cases it was more rapid than in normal individuals. Thus, regardless of whether the patient appeared dehydrated or edematous, the tissues demonstrated a tendency to retain water.

Attempts were also made to measure nitrogen balance in selected patients. While measurements could not be made with the precision necessary to draw conclusions about specific changes in nitrogen metabolism in various body compartments, sufficient data were collected to reach certain general conclusions. Overall balance, as would be expected, was negative. However, the loss of nitrogen was much less than might have been expected—another example of adaptive response by the body, this time in an effort to conserve nitrogen and hence lean body mass.

This chapter, then, presented dramatic evidence, more clearly than ever before, of the body's adaptive response to prolonged semistarvation. In the past few years this adaptive response has come under intensive investigation. Not only have studies been made probing the nature of the metabolic adaptations, including temperature regulation, cardiovascular adaptation, and changes in hormonal regulation, but also studies of tissue and cellular adaptation have begun. Current data strongly suggest that RNA metabolism and protein metabolism at the cellular level undergo a series of "adaptive" changes in prolonged semistarvation and that rehabilitation requires a period of readaptation. The studies of Keys and his collaborators dramatically demonstrated the importance of this adaptive response during the rehabilitative phase of their investigation. The return to normal of the adapted metabolic systems occurs at different rates, especially if refeeding is vigorous. Hence metabolic rate increases rapidly (this was observed also by the Warsaw investigators after dietary carbohydrate supplementation). By contrast, changes in blood volume occur much more slowly. The heart, therefore, suddenly finds itself presented with an increased work load. The result in a number of Keys' patients and in numerous patients treated after World War II and in subsequent famines was congestive heart failure. Another example of this disproportional readaptation is described by the author of this chapter. As the acidosis is corrected, especially if the correction is made very rapidly, hypocalcemia and tetany can be induced.

A careful reading of this chapter sets forth certain cautions about how rehabilitation should be undertaken—lessons that the medical community has learned the hard way through the years. We can only speculate about the number of additional lives that might have been saved had the details of these remarkable studies, carried out under impossible conditions by physicians of the Warsaw ghetto, been widely available before. We believe that their availability now will increase the general knowledge of the metabolic adaptations that occur in semistarvation, will stimulate further research, and will contribute directly to the better care of patients. These were the objectives of the Warsaw investigators when they undertook these studies and we are confident that with the publication in English of this chapter these objectives will be reached.

FOUR Pathophysiology of the Circulatory System in Hunger Disease

Dr. Emil Apfelbaum-Kowalski

with the collaboration of

Dr. Ryszard Pakszwer

Jeanne Zarchi (medical student)

Dr. Ari Heller

Dr. Zdzislaw Askanas

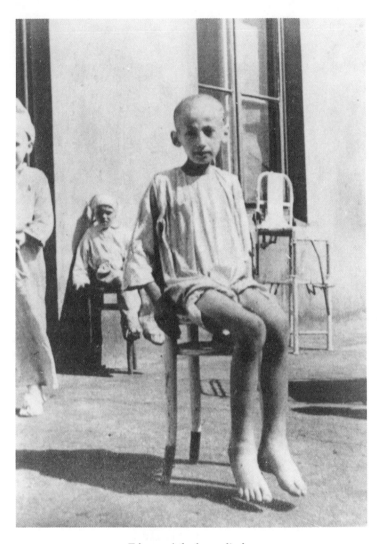

Edema of the lower limbs.

Hunger Disease

Death from long lasting hunger is like a candle burning out slowly. The hungry person becomes lazy, miserly, hoarding the last of his vital energy. His movements are extremely slow and often carefully calculated. The inertia sometimes lasts for days. There is a tendency to lie in a prone position, to feel sleepy, and to maintain silence. Reflexes are inhibited and the psyche is dormant.

In this clinical picture two forces dominate, insufficiency of nutrients and economy of energy. But economizing has its limits. Even a vegetative existence depends on physicochemical reactions which keep the colloidal balance of living cells. Basal metabolism at rest has its ultimate lower limit compatible with life.

Simple calculation shows that in hunger cachexia there must be alterations in the level of basal metabolism at rest. A healthy normal person uses an average of 50 calories per kg of body weight, or about 3000 calories in 24 hours. For many months our patients were eating no more than 10 to 15 calories per kg, or 600 to 800 calories in 24 hours; therefore there was a deficit of 2000 to 2500 calories in 24 hours. From our clinical data we can assume that patients with hunger cachexia lose about 25% of their body weight, thus gaining about 1000 to 1500 calories by burning their own tissues. According to this calculation, a person could survive only 60 to 75 days. However, it was clear from talking to our patients that, without exception, only after several months, and in some cases 1 year, did the symptoms of hunger cachexia appear. We must conclude, therefore, that the organism when confronted by hunger manages its energy balance differently from a normal working man.

The physiological demands of the hungry organism are somehow similar to those of animals hibernating in winter, when only a minimum of energy is used for work and moving around. Otherwise their energy, which comes from burning their own tissues, would not last long.

In this chapter we investigate the mechanism of energy regulation. Our clinical material is unique and cannot be compared with anything so far described in the medical literature, as far as number of cases, duration of hunger, and degree of cachexia.

CLINICAL INVESTIGATIONS OF CARDIOVASCULAR SYMPTOMS

Principles of Physiopathology of the Cardiovascular System

Understanding hunger disease is possible only after consideration of the factors involved in cardiac work, since this work is extremely important in the overall energy metabolism of the organism. Considering only the state of the patients upon examination and studying only the clinical symptoms, we can evaluate the degree to which the organism has been destroyed by hunger, but we need more precise studies to clarify the pathogenesis of the changes that occur during hunger. Precise data on tissue metabolism and on cardiac function allow us to evaluate the functional cardiac disability.

Since in our study we used methods not used by other authors, before discussing hunger cachexia we will explain these new cardiological principles. Cardiac work fulfills the oxygen demands of the tissues and organs. We can calculate the amount of work after having calculated the volume of circulating blood and the circulation time. The volume of circulating blood was determined by the well known color method and circulation time was determined by a method previously described by the first author.

Cardiac work, namely its volume per minute, the amount of blood pumped by heart in one minute, can be expressed by the equation

$$\frac{\text{volume of circulating blood} \times 60}{\text{circulation time}}$$

Example: if volume of blood = 5 liters and circulation time = 30 seconds,

$$cardiac\ work/\text{minute} = \frac{5 \times 60}{30} = 10\ \text{liters}$$

Stroke volume is calculated by dividing the value of cardiac work per minute by the pulse rate. *Example:* if cardiac work = 10 liters and pulse = 80/minute.

$$\text{stroke volume} = \frac{10\ \text{liters}}{80} = 125\ \text{cc}$$

We call the system hemodynamic, since it concerns the volume of circulating blood, cardiac work, and stroke volume, and since these factors express the dynamics of the circulation. This system applies to physiological conditions at rest and at work, expressing the degree of tissue metabolism. Catabolism of tissues is measured by the volume of oxygen used. This volume can be calculated by determining the difference between the amount of oxygen in arterial and the amount in venous blood.

One of the authors (E.A.) devised a method to measure circulation time in capillaries and in tissues. Using this method, we can calculate the degree of activity of tissue metabolism by dividing the volume of used oxygen by the capillary blood circulation time. *Example:* if 5 cc of O_2 were used and time = 10 seconds, the quotient of activity is 5 cc/10 = 0.5.

Our research proved that in a healthy person there is a balance between hemodynamics and metabolism, and that this balance is stable and can be expressed quantitatively. For instance the metabolism at rest in a hemodynamic system is dependent upon the following factors:

1. Volume of circulating blood, 4 to 6 liters, or 75 to 80 cc per kg body weight.
2. Circulation time, 30 to 32 seconds.
3. Cardiac work, 8 to 10 liters.
4. Stroke volume, 80 to 100 cc.

In a metabolic system:

1. Saturation of arterial blood with oxygen is about 95%, or 20 cc in 100 cc of blood.

2. Saturation of venous blood with oxygen is about 60 to 65%, or 15 cc in 100 cc of blood.
3. Arteriovenous difference (oxygen used by tissues) is $\pm$ 4 to 5 cc.
4. Circulation time in capillaries is 9 to 12 seconds.
5. Activity of the periphery = arteriovenous difference/capillary circulation time = 4 to 5/9 to 12 = 0.35 to 0.40.

We have previously demonstrated that in heart failure there is a lack of correlation between the metabolic system, namely, the degree of burning by the tissues, and the hemodynamic system, namely, the volume, the circulation time, and cardiac work. A study of this lack of correlation is essential in understanding the pathogenesis of cardiovascular diseases. We concluded from our studies that often in cases where circulation time is lower than normal, the hemodynamic system is inefficient and cardiac work increases. In many patients an increased volume of circulating blood is also an important factor in cardiac overload.

The abnormal combustion of oxygen in the periphery results in disturbances in cardiovascular circulation and with them poor working conditions for the heart. In most cases in which the use of oxygen by the tissues is increased, the heart is not overloaded because when more oxygen is extracted by the tissues from the blood, the less blood the heart has to pump toward the tissues. In order to explain the lack of energy, the correlation between the metabolic and hemodynamic systems in cardiovascular disease can be divided into several groups. From clinical observations we have found that the poorer the correlation between cardiac action and tissue metabolism, the worse the state of the patient and the worse his prognosis. In most cases of latent circulatory dysfunction there is very poor correlation because of an increased volume of circulating blood or because of changes in the circulation time and heart action or, most often, because of an abnormally increased process of tissue oxygenation. Such results predict serious hypofunction of the circulation and a very serious prognosis.

The observations mentioned above can partly explain the symptoms of circulatory dysfunction. In summary,

1. Cardiac edema is not related to reduced blood flow within tissues.
2. Cyanosis is the result of excessive removal of oxygen from blood and not the result of abnormal oxygenation of arterial blood.
3. Symptoms of passive congestion in the lungs appear together with considerable slowdown of the general blood circulation and some slowdown in the capillaries ("lung barrier").

We now intend to present the techniques used in our study on hunger disease. (The metabolic research had to be interrupted.) Our study concerned the volume of circulating blood, general and tissue connected circulation times, cardiac work per minute, and stroke volume. We studied arterial, venous, and pulse pressure. The degree of tissue metabolism was calculated from the data of resting metabolism, as determined in our clinical material. The data were correlated with clinical observations and electrocardiograms.

Methods Employed in these Studies

1. *Circulation time (authors' method)*. Ten cc of a 1% solution of Congo red dye is injected intravenously into the subject. A second needle rests in the vein for the duration of the experiment and every 2 to 3 seconds a sample is taken into a capillary glass tube. In all, 10 to 20 samples are taken, and time is noted. The capillary tubes are sealed with a Bunsen burner and then centrifuged. The time elapsed between the injection of Congo red and the collecting of the first sample with red stained plasma is the circulation time. Sometimes the red color is doubtful, and addition of one drop of 50% HCl changes the color to blue, confirming the presence of the dye.

2. *Capillary and tissue circulation time (authors' method).* A needle is inserted into the antecubital vein. Another short needle is inserted at a 45° angle into the antecubital artery on the same side. The arterial needle is connected to a syringe containing a 3% solution of Congo red. Slowly 0.25 to 0.35 ml of this dye is injected. The samples are collected from the needle in the vein as in the previous method. The time elapsed between the injection of the dye and the collection of the first sample with colored plasma is the circulation time in the capillaries.

3. *Volume of the circulating blood. Principle.* Dye injected into the vein has the greatest concentration at 4 minutes after the injection. The degree of red coloring is the measure of the volume of blood. The greater the volume, the paler the color.

Method. The patient is resting in a prone position. We collect 10 cc of blood to obtain a 0 second time sample of plasma; then we inject 10 cc of a 1% solution of Congo red. In exactly 4 minutes we collect another 10 cc of blood. The tubes with blood contained just a pinch of calcium oxalate. After spinning for 30 seconds we read the color on a Pulfrich spectrophotometer. Before separating the plasma we read the levels of RBCs and plasma to calculate the percent of their respective volumes. With a Pasteur pipette the plasma is transferred to the glass containers of the spectrophotometer and read using filter S50. Each concentration equals the negative logarithm of the number read. Knowing the amount of injected dye and its concentration, we calculated the volume of circulating plasma. Knowing the percent relationship of RBCs and plasma, we can calculate the volume of circulating blood; dividing it by body weight, we obtain the volume of blood per kilogram of body weight.

4. *Volume per minute.* This ratio is calculated from the hemodynamic formula.

5. *Determination of basal metabolism.* The volume of oxygen inhaled in 1 minute is determined by using the Plantefol apparatus. The patient breathes through a tube into a glass bottle which collects the exhaled air. Using the connected gas meter,

we can determine the volume of air inhaled in 1 minute. With an endiometer we can calculate volume % and carbon dioxide in each collected sample. By multiplying volume % of oxygen by volume of inhaled air, the volume of oxygen inhaled in 1 minute is determined. The respiratory quotient equals CO_2/O_2. Basal metabolism can be calculated from appropriate tables considering body weight, age, and sex.

6. *Oscillometry.* Oscillometric fluctuations at rest and at work were calculated with a Recklinhausen oscillometer according to well known principles. Bedridden patients worked by sitting and lying down.

7. *Venous pressure.* This was determined by using a manometric clock and Ringer filled manometer. Work was carried out as previously described.

8. *Electrocardiography.* An electrocardiogram connected to a Siemens galvanometer was used.

CLINICAL STUDY OF THE CARDIOVASCULAR SYSTEM IN HUNGER DISEASE

For our study we tried to obtain homogeneous material and clean hunger disease patients. Therefore we excluded all cases complicated by other diseases. It was sometimes very difficult, especially with people with anergic tuberculosis, which in cachexic patients shows no symptoms. Our patients were 16 to 30 years old, most of them from refugee centers, and some from the streets, who were at the limit of cachexia. They had been consuming about 800 calories daily for a long time. Many of them could hardly move, and even those that still could preferred to stay motionless in bed. They were all placed in one ward for hunger disease. The research on the pathodynamics of the cardiovascular system concerns mostly the volume of blood and cardiac work.

Blood Volume

Of the 18 cases of cachexia we examined, in only two cases was the blood volume in the normal range (4 to 6 liters). The reduced volume in the other 16 cases was usually at the lower physiological limits. However, in five cases it was markedly reduced (2.39, 1.74, 2.62, 2.51, 2.79). The average was 3.7 liters.

It would seem from these values that in hunger cachexia it is a biological necessity to reduce blood volume in order to minimize cardiac work. But this is only an illusion, because when one considers that the body weight of these patients is only 50% of normal (the average was 32 kg) one realizes that when calculating the blood volume per kilogram of body weight the volume of blood is actually *increased*.

Under physiological conditions the relationship of blood volume to body weight is quite stable, between 80 and 100 cc per kg. In three cases of hunger disease it was at the upper limit of normal. In 13 cases it was much higher than 100 cc per kg. The average of all 16 cases was 114 cc. Since most of the patients had edema, the actual volume would have been even greater if body weight had been expressed after deducting the weight of water contained in the edema.

The increased volume of circulating blood is a very important factor in the pathodynamics of the cardiovascular system in hunger cachexia because the poorly nourished cardiac muscle has to work even harder than in a normal individual. The data quoted here corresponded only to resting basal metabolism. However, considering the way of life of a person with hunger cachexia we feel that this is the most valid comparison to normal people which can be made. Movement and physical work markedly increase blood volume under physiological conditions. In hunger cachexia movement and physical work cannot affect the blood volume very much because there is very little blood in the cisterns. Therefore, during work the volume of blood may be lower than in normal people.

Circulation time is an important mechanism regulating the

work of a heart overloaded because of an increased volume of blood. In 18 examined cases of hunger cachexia (Table 1) the blood velocity was determined by the method described above and found to be very low. The normal velocity is 32 seconds; in two of our cases it was 42 to 45 seconds (cases 10 through 12). Some cases were as slow as 80 seconds (cases 2 and 9). Marked slowing of the velocity occurs also in other types of cardiovascular disease. Therefore, this symptom is not pathognomonic for hunger cachexia. On the contrary, it is a compensatory mechanism to diminish cardiac work. From our hemodynamic index it can be readily seen that cardiac work represents the relationship between the volume of blood and its circulation time. The longer the time, the less the work for the heart.

It is clear from looking at Table 1 that minute volume in normal people at rest is 8 to 10 liters and that in hunger cachexia it is markedly reduced. In cases 1 and 2 it was 2.4 liters and 1.4 liters respectively. In other cases it was between 3 and 6 liters, with an average of 4 liters, which is 50% of normal. Figure 1 presents the pathology of cardiac work in hunger disease. The left column represents normal conditions; 5 liters of circulating blood runs through the body in 30 seconds or 10 liters per minute (horizontal lines). The right column represents hunger cachexia. Cardiac output in one minute (55 seconds) equals only 5 liters, almost half as much as normal.

One of the features of the clinical picture in hunger disease is the predominance of the vagus system over the sympathetic system as expressed, for example, in the slow cardiac systole. This is a fundamental abnormality because in most situations connected with reduced basal metabolism the tonus of the vagus system is increased. In evaluating the cardiac symptoms in hunger disease the slow pulse can be considered a positive feature in the economy of cardiac work because in spite of the reduced cardiac output, stroke volume is increased and cardiac muscle repolarization is better during ventricular diastole. It is obvious from Table 1 that the slowing down of the pulse was really considerable; in 50% of the cases it was 48 to 54 per minute. In

TABLE 1   BLOOD CIRCULATION VELOCITY AND CARDIAC WORK IN HUNGER CACHEXIA

Case	Age (years)	Weight (kg)	Volume of Blood Total (liters)	Volume of Blood Per kg (ml)	Velocity (sec)	Cardiac Work Minute Volume (liters)	Cardiac Work Pulse	Cardiac Work Systolic Volume (ml)	Volume % RBC	Volume % Plasma
1	42	41.5	2.39	57	58	2.47	81	30	35	65
2	25	35.5	1.74	49	73	1.43	87	16	26.6	73.4
3	30	30	4.54	150	55	4.96	54	92	26	74
4	19	30.85	3.97	128	65	3.67	48	76	28	72
5	26	35.25	3.1	87	54	3.45	51	67	33	67
6	16	35	6.14	175	59	6.24	54	115	26	74
7	27	26	3.13	118	68	2.76	51	54	26	74
8	29	24	2.62	109	59	2.67	75	35	32	68
9	26	33	5.21	157	80	3.90	66	59	49	51
10	18	26.6	2.51	94	42	3.58	60	60	29	71
11	38	30.4	3.21	84	45	4.27	63	67	27.7	72.3
12	14	25.9	2.79	108	43	3.90	51	76	30	70
13	20	33.3	4.08	122	65	3.70	78	47	32	68
14	22	41.5	4.21	101	43	5.80	48	120	35.5	64.5
15	26	31	3.50	113	55	3.83	66	58	34	66
16	32	40	6.50	162	48	8.10	48	171	35	65
17	40	30	3.60	120	54	4.0	66	60	37	63
18	38	30	3.51	116	55	3.82	52	73	24	76
Average		32.2	3.7	114	57	4.0	61	70	31.4	68.3
Physiologic		—	4–6	80–100	32	8–10	72–84	90–100	45	55

Hunger Disease

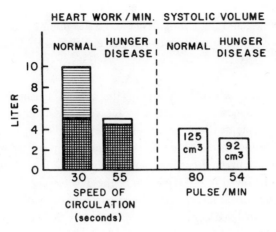

Figure 1   Heart work per minute and systolic volume.

other patients it was slightly higher and only in four cases was it normal.

In comparison to pulse rate, the systolic volume was only slightly lower than normal, 70 cc (normal being 90 to 100 cc), but the difference is not as large as the difference in minute volume.

In Figure 1 cardiac work (left side of figure) is twice as great in the normal heart as it is in the hearts of patients with hunger disease. Stroke volume in hunger disease is almost normal—92 cc as compared to 125 cc in the normal heart (right side of figure).

From this study we can conclude that the diminished circulation time and the diminished heart rate make it easier for the heart to supply blood to the tissues.

Our EKG studies were conducted on 12 cases, both at rest and after exertion (15 situps in 30 seconds in bed). Studying the QRS complex we see

1. Regular, slow sinus rhythm.
2. Very low voltage.
3. Normal ventricular system.
4. T waves of low amplitude in all leads, occasionally inverted.

5. Prolonged and frequently depressed ST segment.
6. Almost no difference between the exertional EKG and the resting EKG.

Ischemia and easy exhaustion of the undernourished cardiac muscle are suggested, especially by the very low voltage and the ST segment depression. Low amplitude T waves also demonstrate ischemic cardiac muscle. The long T wave suggests that in an undernourished cardiac muscle repolarization is effective, since it is believed that the pattern of the T wave depends on the speed of disappearance of functional currents in cardiac muscle. The fact that the EKG does not change after the exertion demonstrates that the heart is working at the limits of its capabilities and exercise does not affect its dynamic action.

The EKG considered together with the cardiac work described above shows that in hunger disease conditions are abnormal. Exertion in a normal person results in an EKG with a rapid sinus rhythm, shortening of the duration of particular segments and waves, and increased electric or ionic activity in cardiac muscle as measured by increased voltage. Dynamic reflexes disappear in hunger cachexia and the adaptive cardiac regulation becomes "fixed." The basic work of the heart cannot be changed. Even at rest the heart is really in a stage of heart failure because of its low electric energy and low voltage.

Capillary circulation time and oxygen consumption. Even at rest the basal metabolism of patients with hunger disease, as measured by the small amount of oxygen used per minute, shows a decline. As shown in Table 2, under normal conditions the volume of oxygen varies from 200 to 250 cc. From our previous research we also know that in normal individuals the circulation time in the capillaries is 9 to 14 seconds.

Table 3 demonstrates the changes in hunger disease. The volume of oxygen varies from 100 to 140 cc, half of normal. In addition, basal metabolism could be as low as -36% with an average of -22.5%. Regardless of the degree of cachexia, the volume of oxygen consumed is never less than 100 cc. Obvi-

TABLE 2   VELOCITY OF BLOOD CIRCULATION IN
CAPILLARIES AND OXYGEN METABOLISM IN NORMAL
TISSUES

Case	Age (years)	Weight (kg)	Sex	Velocity (sec)	Basal Metabolism (%)	Oxygen Volume (ml/min)
1	38	62	Male	9	+2	202
2	18	59	Male	11	+4	189
3	24	69	Male	14	0	254
4	28	51	Male	10	−3	195
5	34	54	Female	13	+1	222
6	19	55	Female	9	0	199
Average				11	+1	243

ously this is the minimum necessary for survival. We were not able to do any further studies on blood oxygenation. One indication of decreased oxygenation by the tissues is the rarity of cyanosis in even the most severe cases of hunger cachexia. This observation demonstrates that the volume of deoxygenated hemoglobin does not exceed Lundsgaard's "threshold of cyanosis." In far advanced anemia there is no cyanosis because of an inadequate amount of hemoglobin, and, as we have discovered, the

TABLE 3   VELOCITY OF BLOOD CIRCULATION IN
CAPILLARIES AND OXYGEN METABOLISM IN HUNGER
CACHEXIA

Case	Age (years)	Weight (kg)	Sex	Velocity (sec)	Basal Metabolism (%)	Oxygen Volume (ml/min)
1	25	35.5	Female	42	−33.7	105
2	30	30	Female	29	−9.7	137
3	19	31	Female	—	−36.1	124
4	26	35	Female	32	−12.1	140
5	27	26	Female	33	−21	108
6	29	24	Female	—	−29.7	98
7	18	26.6	Female	28	−15	125
8	18	—	Female	24	—	—
9	21	—	Female	18	—	—
Average				29	−22.5	119

degree of chlorosis in hunger cachexia is not high enough to re-sult in cyanosis since there is an adequate amount of oxygen to exceed the "cyanosis threshold."

Reduced tissue catabolism is accompanied by slower blood circulation in the capillaries as shown in Table 3. Normally capillary circulation time is 9 to 14 seconds. In hunger disease it slows to 18 to 42 seconds with an average of 29 seconds.

TABLE 4   OSCILLATION FLUCTUATION AT REST AND AFTER WORK

Case	Age (years)	Sex	150		140		130		120		110		100	
			Rest	Work	Rest	Work	Rest	Work	Rest	Work	Rest	Work	Rest	Wo
1	23		—	—	—	½	½	1	1½	1½	2	2½	2½	3
2	31	Male	—	—	—	½	—	¾	¾	1½	1½	2½	2½	3
3	33	Male	—	—	—	—	1	¾	1½	2	2½	3½	4	4½
4	25	Male	—	1	1	2½	1½	3	2	1½	2½	4½	4	5
5	20	Male	—	¾	¾	1	1	1½	2½	2½	3	4½	4	5
6	19	Male	—	—	—	¾	1	1	1½	1½	2	2	2½	2½
7	25	Male	0	¾	0	¾	¾	1	1	1	2	2½	3	3½
8	24	Male	—	—	0	¾	0	1	1	2	1½	3½	2	4½
9	29	Male	—	—	—	—	0	¾	¾	1½	1½	2½	2	3
10	33	Male	0	1½	¾	3	2	4	3	4½	4½	5½	5½	6½

TABLE 5   OSCILLATION FLUCTUATION AT REST AND AFTER WORK

Case	Age (years)	Sex	130		120		110		100		90		80	
			Rest	Work	Rest	Work	Rest	Work	Rest	Work	Rest	Work	Rest	W
1	22	Female	—	—	—	½	—	½	½	1	1½	2	2½	2
2	18	Female	—	—	—	—	—	—	—	—	0	½	½	1
3	33	Female	—	—	½	¾	1¼	2	2	3	3	4	3½	4
4	30	Female	—	—	—	—	—	—	½	1	1½	2	2	3
5	29	Female	—	—	—	—	—	—	—	—	½	—	¾	
6	25	Female	—	½	—	¾	¾	¾	½	½	—	—	—	
7	14	Female	—	—	—	—	—	—	—	—	—	—	1	1
8	16	Female	—	—	—	—	—	—	—	—	¾	1	1	1
9	30	Female	—	—	—	—	—	2¼	1½	2½	2½	3½	3	4
10	18	Female	—	—	—	—	—	—	—	—	1½	1½	2	
11	26	Female	—	—	—	—	—	—	—	—	½	½	1	

HEMODYNAMICS AT REST AND AFTER EXERTION

Oscillometric and Arterial Pressure

The amount of work accomplished by the heart depends partly on arterial and venous pressure. We examined 10 normal cases (Table 4) and 11 cases of hunger cachexia (Table 5) at rest

NORMAL PEOPLE (mm Hg)

										Blood Pressure					
90		80		70		60		50		Systolic		Diastolic		Median	
Rest	Work	Rest	Work	Rest	Work	Rest	Work	Rest	Work	Rest	Work	Rest	Work	Rest	Work
	3½	1½	2½	1	1½	½	1	—	—	125	130	80	80	90	95
	4½	4½	5½	4	4	1½	2	—	—	120	135	60	60	80	75
1½	5	4	4½	1½	4	1½	2	—	1	125	125	65	55	95	100
1½	4	2	2½	1	1½	—	1½	—	—	140	150	85	80	95	100
	6	5½	6	4½	5½	1½	4½	—	2½	135	150	65	55	80	85
1½	3	2	2½	1	2	—	—	—	—	130	135	60	60	90	85
	5	6½	7	5	7	—	—	—	—	130	150	75	70	80	90
	3½	3½	4	1	2	—	—	—	—	125	140	65	65	80	100
½	2½	1	2	—	—	—	—	—	—	120	130	70	75	100	105
	7½	3	6	2	3	—	—	—	—	140	150	70	70	85	90

HUNGER CACHEXIA (mm Hg)

										Blood Pressure					
70		60		50		40		30		Systolic		Diastolic		Median	
Rest	Work	Rest	Work	Rest	Work	Rest	Work	Rest	Work	Rest	Work	Rest	Work	Rest	Work
	3½	1½	3	—	1½	—	—	—	—	95	100	60	45	70	65
¾	1½	1	1½	—	¾	½	½	—	—	70	90	40	40	55	60
½	4	2½	3	¼	1½	1	1	¾	½	110	115	40	45	75	75
½	—	2½	1½	—	1	—	—	—	—	95	100	75	80	50	60
¾	¼	¼	—	—	—	—	—	—	—	Not to be measured					
¼	2	1½	2½	1	1½	0	1	—	—	80	80	50	40	65	65
½	1½	1	1	1	¾	—	—	—	—	90	90	65	60	75	80
½	4	2½	2½	1½	1	1	½	—	—	100	105	40	55	75	80
½	2¼	1½	2	½	½	—	—	—	—	85	80	50	65	75	70
	1½	2¾	2½	2½	2½	—	1½	—	—	80	80	40	45	55	65

and after exertion in order to study the circulatory changes in hunger.

It is known that the oscillations measure systolic cardiac work, filling of the arteries, volume of the circulating blood, and arterial wall elasticity. The turgor of tissues and their functional condition also affect the oscillation.

In 10 healthy young people that we examined the data on oscillation, on systolic, diastolic, and average blood pressure (Vaquez) were almost identical. After work (15 situps in bed) we observed

1. An increase of about 15 mm Hg in systolic pressure.
2. An increase of about 5 mm Hg in mean pressure.
3. Slight lowering of the diastolic pressure.
4. An increase in pulse wave amplitude from 10 to 15 mm Hg.

These changes after work suggest a sudden increase in systolic volume, considerable filling of arteries and capillaries, and increased turgor of the working tissues due to their increased metabolism. Figure 2 shows an interrupted line for work and a solid line for rest (left side normal subjects; right side patients with hunger disease).

In patients with hunger cachexia at rest we see that

1. Systolic arterial pressure is much lower than in normal people. It is 80 to 115 mm Hg.
2. Diastolic pressure is slightly lower.

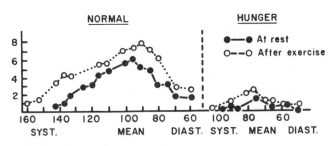

Figure 2   Blood pressures at rest and after exercise.

3. Pulse wave is reduced.
4. Oscillation fluctuations are much smaller than in normal people.

In very severe hunger cachexia, oscillation fluctuations are minimal (see Table 5 and right side of Figure 2). In some patients it was impossible even to measure blood pressure. The findings after exercise are interesting:

1. Only rarely do systolic and diastolic pressures increase.
2. The pulse wave does not change.
3. Fluctuations are fixed, with almost identical curves at rest and at work (Figure 2, right side).

Studies of the arterial system reflect findings similar to those in the hemodynamic system. Minimal fluctuations and lowering of the systolic pressure suggest diminished cardiac work. "Fixed" curves after work demonstrate a very limited, almost nonexistent, effect of work as a stimulus for the cardiovascular system. Even slightly elevated oxidative processes in the working tissues are not paralleled by an adaptive cardiac response. Clinical observations of the apathetic behavior of the patients confirm these observations.

Venous pressure was examined in five normal subjects and in seven cases of hunger cachexia (Table 6). Under normal conditions it was 12 to 14 mm Hg. After work it would increase by 3 to 4 mm Hg. In hunger cachexia it was much lower, 9 to 12 mm Hg. After effort the increase was only 1 to 2 mm Hg. In two cases (7 and 10) venous pressure was very high, similar to what is usually seen in cardiac failure. In hunger cachexia the venous system is also relatively unresponsive.

DISCUSSION

Our research on the vascular system in hunger disease had the following objectives: to determine the type and essence of the

TABLE 6 VENOUS PRESSURE AT REST AND AFTER WORK IN NORMAL PEOPLE AND HUNGER CACHEXIA

Case	Age (years)	Sex	Venous Pressure		Pulse	
			Rest	Work	Rest	Work
		Normal				
1	25	Male	14	18	75	90
2	31	Male	14	11	63	84
3	18	Female	12	16	72	78
4	23	Female	12	15	70	84
5	28	Male	13	16	72	88
		Hunger Cachexia				
6	22	Female	9	8	63	60
7	25	Female	21	19	88	88
8	14	Female	12	12	57	60
9	16	Female	12	13	99	105
10	30	Female	21	19	63	72
11	18	Female	10	10	69	76
12	26	Female	11	12	66	69

pathodynamic symptoms, to determine the relationship of these symptoms to tissue metabolism, and to determine the type and essence of the malfunction of the cardiovascular system seen during hunger disease of long duration. The homogeneity of our results and the good fit among separate links in the chain of pathological symptoms make it easier to synthesize the findings in this clinically new problem.

Our research clearly demonstrates that the syndrome of persistent hunger is a definite pathological entity. Metabolism is altered in specific ways and takes on a new form. Metabolic changes and changes within the cardiovascular system that have not been previously reported occur during the struggle against hunger. Although many studies have been carried out before, the hunger was never so prolonged as to lead to cachexia and death, and the clinical material was never so numerous.

THE BASIC NATURE OF THE CARDIOVASCULAR MALFUNCTION IN HUNGER CACHEXIA

The body suffering from prolonged hunger is operating under a large and constant caloric deficiency, since the energy expended is not replaced. The negative energy balance reduces the physiological activities of the patients to a minimum (vita minima).

The cardiovascular system, and indeed all the other organs, must adjust to these general conditions of energy. The economy and the extent of such adjustment are in part determined by the degree and duration of hunger. Our work proved that this adjustment is not complete and that it is accompanied by certain pathological changes. The volume of circulating blood, when calculated on a body weight basis, was increased in 90% of the cases, which was contrary to our expectations. In advanced hunger cachexia the increase was considerable. Such an increase is obviously not to the advantage of the heart, since cardiac work must be increased to cope with the increased volume of blood. How can we explain the atrophy of tissues and organs and the increased amount of blood, which would tend to throw energy metabolism even further out of balance? The increase in blood volume consists of an increase in water in blood. The volume of plasma increases to 70 to 75% in comparison with 55% under normal circumstances. This is the result of the direction of the flow of water. Clinical studies on these patients also demonstrated the high degree of water in both plasma and RBCs in hunger disease.

The sum of the increased volume of circulating blood and the amount of water in RBCs and plasma is the measure of the amount of water flowing from the tissues into the vascular system. The surplus of water in the blood creates a vicious cycle which forces the circulation to push through a surplus of blood. The limited calories available, which are insufficient to supply tissue energy, become even more limited as a result of the dilution of the blood. The excessive dilution of the blood reduces its value as a carrier of nutritive substances and therefore the vascular system is forced to supply more of this low value blood to the hungry tissues and organs.

A similar mechanism prevails with respect to oxygen. The reduced number of circulating RBCs and the reduced amount of circulating hemoglobin, which results from a barrier in the bone marrow, and the waterlogged RBCs all contribute to inadequate oxygenation of the tissues, even though their requirements are not very large. Because of its poor oxygenation, blood has to reach the tissues in excess. As Eppinger has reported, the flow of water from atrophying tissues makes the tissue oxygenation even more difficult.

These factors result in the circulation of an increased volume of diluted blood. This situation is incompatible with normal cardiac function. But in spite of this stress, complete breakdown of the cardiovascular system rarely occurs in hunger cachexia. From these studies we have gained some insight into how the cardiovascular system copes with this shaky dynamic balance. All of the patients examined had very long circulation times, which decreases the cardiac work per minute, improving the dynamics of the circulation and helping to regenerate the poorly nourished cardiac muscle. Our results indicate that about 40% of the cases with cardiac malfunction show a slowing down of the circulation. In spite of diminished cardiac output, the stroke volume in hunger cachexia is only minimally lowered. This can be explained by the slower pulse rate (50 to 60 per minute). Concomitant with the general slowing of the circulation, the circulation in the capillaries and tissues is also slowed down. We cannot exclude the possibility that prolongation of the passage of RBCs through the capillaries and tissues facilitates oxidation and gas diffusion.

CIRCULATORY DYSFUNCTION AND TISSUE METABOLISM

Diminished consumption of oxygen and lowering of the basal metabolism demonstrate that the catabolism of the tissues and organs is limited. Clinical observations and the study of EKG tracings show that the cardiac muscle, even at rest, is ischemic. The low voltage, the low amplitude of T waves, and in many cases the depressed ST segment confirm the above observations. The inadequate metabolism of the cardiac muscle affects its efficiency. Under physiological conditions, oxygenation of tissues and organs is markedly increased by exertion. By contrast, in hunger cachexia metabolism is almost identical at rest and after exertion. To our knowledge this lack of change is unique. In normal individuals and in patients suffering from a variety of illnesses exertion increases oxygenation and cardiac work, but in a chronically hungry patient there is no change after exercise because of a lack of cardiac adaptation. Heart rate, stroke volume, systolic pressure, pulse wave, and oscillations remain the same. Comparing the EKGs of different patients, we notice identical tracings at rest and after exertion. Sinus rhythm is not accelerated, voltage is not increased, and conductivity of particular segments of the EKG remains the same. Clinical observations confirm the fact that exertion in a chronically hungry organism is insignificant. There is no difference between movement and rest. Even approaching death does not affect metabolism; the limits between living and dying are blurred. The cardiovascular system approaching the last moments does not change its work; the motor of life stops not because of a dissociation between particular parts but because of a lack of fuel.

ENDOCRINE AND AUTONOMIC SYSTEMS AND THEIR ROLE IN ENERGY METABOLISM

As with all other organs, the glands show symptoms of dysfunction. For example:

1. The low basal metabolism in the tissues and organs and the lack of reaction to external stimuli can be explained by reduced function of the thyroid and pituitary glands. Even

the type of cachexia and the slow response of different atrophying organs resemble Simmonds' disease.

2. Skin pigmentation, low blood pressure, low body temperature, low resistance, especially to tuberculosis, slight sexual reversal (facial hair in cachexic girls or in young boys) suggest dysfunction of the adrenal cortex.

3. Cessation of menstruation and reduced libido may be connected with dysfunction of the ovaries.

4. Osteomalacia and osteoporosis suggest dysfunction of the parathyroid glands.

5. The pancreas is the only endocrine organ without obvious signs of dysfunction.

We believe that insulin is being produced adequately. The body does not need much insulin because the amount of ingested carbohydrates, which regulates the production of this hormone, is small. We believe that in carbohydrate metabolism the proinsulin system predominates over insulin antagonists. Low blood sugar levels can be explained by the small amounts of ingested carbohydrates in hunger disease, partially diluted blood, and exaggerated affinity for sugar from organs deprived of glycogen. Clinically the lack of hypoglycemic symptoms would also exclude a surplus of insulin in the blood. The abnormalities in the endocrine system in hunger cachexia suggest that these glands play an important role in sparing cardiovascular work. This is particularly true for the autonomic system. In spite of reduced autonomic activity in hunger cachexia there is a predominance of economizing forces, namely, the vagus, over the sympathetic system. This predominance can be seen during cardiovascular work, as exemplified by slow pulse, slow circulation time, weak reaction to exertion, low level of arterial pressure, and slow repolarization of the cardiac muscle as seen in the EKG pattern.

ESSENCE AND TYPE OF CARDIOVASCULAR DYSFUNCTION IN HUNGER CACHEXIA

Since in hunger cachexia the cardiovascular system cannot function normally and only with great difficulty does it take care of basal metabolism, we consider that latent cardiovascular insufficiency occurs in cachexia.

Clinically the symptoms of cardiac dysfunction in hunger disease are different from those seen in patients with the usual kind of cardiovascular dysfunction. The following forms of dysfunction were observed in hunger cachexia:

1. There is no passive hyperemia of organs. On the contrary, they are atrophying and bloodless as shown by pathological examination.
2. There is no passive hyperemia in the pulmonary circulation. On the contrary, there is hypoventilation of the lungs, ischemia, and a clinical picture called decreased pulmonary compliance (Orlowski and Gorecki).
3. Increased urinary output, low specific gravity of the urine, and a lack of the characteristic formed elements in the urine exclude the possibility of passive renal congestion.
4. The small size of the liver demonstrates the small volume of blood in this organ.
5. The edema is quite different from that seen in normal cardiovascular dysfunction. It is pale, randomly distributed, and does not increase after a day's work.
6. Cyanosis is observed only occasionally because of the low level of tissue oxygenation and the oxygen deficit in the circulating hemoglobin.
7. Dyspnea is a very rare symptom even after effort. The slow superficial breathing suggests reduced lung ventilation.
8. After a work stimulus there is no increase in pulse rate, arterial pressure remains the same, and venous pressure remains low.

In some respects there are similarities between the abnormalities in the hemodynamics of hunger disease and other types of cardiovascular dysfunction. In both, slowing of the circulation is balanced by a surplus of circulating blood and a diminished work per minute of the heart. But the tissue oxygen metabolism is different. In simple dysfunction of the cardiovascular system the oxygenation in the tissues is increased and basal metabolism is often increased. Frank dissociation between the increased metabolism and the limited ability to increase cardiovascular work will result in acute or chronic cardiac failure.

In hunger cachexia oxygen metabolism is quite different. Tissue oxidation is diminished and conservation of energy is a positive factor which reduces the work load of the circulation. However, the heart cannot efficiently pump the blood, which contains a surplus of water and is deficient in nutrients and oxygen to adequately supply the needs of all organs including cardiac muscle.

In summary, the clinical picture and pathogenesis of cardiovascular dysfunction in hunger cachexia demonstrate a specific type of hypofunction. The difficulty of coping with effort under these conditions is due not to the lack of correlation between cardiac work and tissue metabolism, but rather to the very limited energy of the organism.

CONCLUSIONS

The following observations were made on people with hunger cachexia. In 18 cases, metabolism at rest, volume of circulating blood, general and tissue circulation time, cardiac output, stroke volume, and volume % of RBCs and serum were measured. Oscillation was measured in 10 normal subjects and 11 patients at rest and after work and arterial and venous pressures were measured in five normal subjects and seven patients. Electrocardiographic studies were performed in 12 patients. The following methods were used:

1. Dye method with Congo red for determination of volume of circulating blood and general and tissue circulation velocity. Cardiac work per minute and stroke volume were calculated from the hemodynamic formula.
2. Work per minute = volume of circulating blood/circulation time.
3. Stroke volume = work per minute/pulse rate.
4. Oscillometry (Recklinhausen).
5. Pantefol apparatus for measurement of basal (resting) metabolism and oxygen utilization per minute.
6. Electrocardiography (Siemens).

We reached the following conclusions from the combined metabolic and clinical observations:

1. The volume of blood per kilogram of body weight is increased because of increased hydration of the serum (probably secondary to transfer of water from disintegrating tissues), the small amount of nutrients in blood, and the inadequate amount of circulating RBCs and hemoglobin. To fulfill the caloric and oxygen demands of tissues there should be an increased amount of blood.
2. General and tissue circulation slows down. This factor balances the surplus of blood in the tissues and probably facilitates the oxydation process.
3. Cardiac work per minute is reduced.
4. Since the pulse rate is slower, stroke volume is only slightly reduced.
5. Examining EKG at rest and after exertion, we observe slow sinus rhythm, low voltage, prolonged ST segment, T waves of low amplitude, depressed ST segment, and identical tracing at rest and after exertion.
6. The clinical data, the low basal metabolism, and the EKG findings lead us to conclude that even at rest cardiac muscle is lacking in oxygen and functionally damaged, repolarization of cardiac muscle is efficient, and the adaptive cardiac regulation becomes "fixed."

7. Oscillation is minimal and does not increase after exertion. There is a reduction in arterial and venous pressure and a reduced pulse wave, and exertion did not affect these results. Thus work of the cardiovascular system is very limited, which agrees with the clinical finding in hunger cachexia.

8. Reduced pulse rate, reduced circulatory velocity, weak response to effort, low arterial blood pressure, and an extended period of repolarization of cardiac muscle when combined with the clinical observations suggest the prevalence of vagal tonus over sympathetic tonus.

9. In hunger cachexia there is latent circulatory hypofunction. In comparing these findings with normal circulatory dysfunctions we conclude that the dysfunction in hunger cachexia represents a separate pathologic entity. Clinically it differs from the usual types of cardiac failure. Instead of passive congestion of the heart, liver, lungs, and kidneys, in hunger cachexia these organs have an inadequate blood supply. In addition the localization of the edema is not characteristic for normal circulatory dysfunction.

Pathophysiologically the dysfunction in hunger edema differs from the usual types of cardiac failure. In the circulatory dysfunction of hunger cachexia, as in other types of dysfunction, there is an increase in circulating blood volume, and a low circulation time or decreased heart work, but in the usual cardiac dysfunction oxygenation of tissues is increased. In addition, in other types of cardiac failure, during exertion there is a dissociation between tissue metabolism and increased work of the heart. In cardiac dysfunction caused by hunger cachexia, oxygen metabolism is very low and remains at the level of basal metabolism even after exertion.

EDITOR'S COMMENTS

Myron Winick, M.D.

The studies described in this chapter demonstrate what an imaginative and disciplined investigator can do even with extremely limited equipment and supplies. The chapter begins with a theoretical discussion of the forces that determine the adaptation of the cardiovascular system in hunger disease. The major pressures on the circulatory system are due to a lack of nutrients and a lowering of body metabolism. The authors point out that by simple arithmetic, one can calculate that an individual surviving on a typical Warsaw ghetto diet could survive for only 60 to 75 days if the metabolic rate remained at its usual level. Since all of their patients and indeed most of the population had survived much longer before they ever showed symptoms of hunger disease, one could assume that the basal metabolic rate drops. The authors compare what is occurring in hunger disease to what occurs during hibernation in certain mammals, a comparison which, although not strictly analogous, is still made today.

In order to evaluate the changes that occurred in the circulation, a number of methods which were new at the time were employed. The authors carefully describe the methods employed and derive the equations that were used to calculate cardiac work and stroke volume. In order to determine these, the volume of circulating blood, the circulation time, and the pulse rate had to be measured. These were sophisticated methods for any research protocol in 1940, and under the prevalent conditions it is truly amazing that they could be carried out. In addition to these measurements, an attempt was made to study the rate of "tissue catabolism" by determining the amount of oxygen used by a tissue. This was measured by calculating the difference between arterial and capillary oxygen content. The rate of oxygen consumption by the tissues could then be determined if the capillary circulation time was determined. The author therefore derived a method for determining capillary circulation time. Thus the circulation could be divided into two systems: the hemodynamic system, which reflected alterations in blood volume, circulation time, cardiac work, and stroke volume, and the "metabolic system," which reflected alterations in oxygen saturation of arterial and venous blood and the differences in their saturation, as well as capillary circulation time and "peripheral activity," which was defined as the arteriovenous difference divided by the capillary circulation time. Dr. Apfelbaum's previous research had established normal values and had determined some of the changes accompanying various forms of heart failure. He points out that in these studies, the larger the discrepancy between these two systems the poorer the prognosis.

The next section describes in detail the various methods employed in making the actual measurements. This is a very important section, since it not only allows us to evaluate the results obtained but also demonstrates the great care and precision that had to be employed in order to obtain valid results. For example, circulation time was measured by dye dilution using Congo red. Two needles had to be inserted into the antecubital vein, the first to inject the dye, and the second, presumably distal to the first, to collect samples every 2 to 3 seconds. Capillary circulation time was determined by injecting a more concentrated solution of Congo red into the antecubital artery and sampling repeatedly from the antecubital vein. Blood volume was measured again by dye dilution 4 minutes after an intravenous injection of Congo red, the time previously determined necessary for the dye to reach equilibrium and maximum concentration. The BMR was determined by measuring the volume of oxygen inhaled in 1 minute and the amount of CO_2 exhaled during the same period. The equipment used for these measurements was the standard used at that time and was designed on principles still used today. The RQ was then calculated as CO_2/O_2, and BMR was derived from appropriate tables using age, sex, and body weight. Blood pressure and venous pressure measurements and electrocardiograms were all carried out by standard methods in the resting state and after exercise (bedridden patients worked by sitting up and lying down).

Thus, in order to obtain the results they desired, these investigators not only employed the techniques most current at that time but also developed their own techniques when an established method was not available. Some of the techniques, for example, the intraarterial injection, were not without risk to the patient. However, the authors obviously felt that the potential benefits to science far outweighed the risks involved, especially under the prevailing conditions. It is hard to find fault with their position.

Using the methods outlined above, the authors report their results and then develop their theories of the pathophysiology of the circulatory changes that occur in hunger disease.

Measurements of blood volume revealed a slight reduction in total circulating blood. However, this reduction was far less than the reduction in body weight, so that the blood volume per kilogram of body weight was significantly increased. The authors point out that these measurements were made at rest and that the increase in circulating blood volume which accompanies exercise may not occur in these patients. They conclude that this increased blood volume, though part of the adaptive response to hunger, places an extra strain on the heart.

The circulation time was found to be markedly increased in these patients, averaging 57 seconds compared to 32 seconds in normal individuals (see Table 2). Keys and co-workers did not actually measure circulation time but do cite these results, pointing out the crude nature of the method employed. Although the absolute times differ with this method from those obtained with the more accurate methods subsequently in use, the relative difference and the ultimate conclusion stand. Circulation time is markedly increased in semistarvation.

From these measurements and the pulse rate, minute volume is calculated. The authors conclude that it is markedly reduced in hunger disease (from 8 to 10 liters in normal individuals to an average of 4 liters in hunger disease (Table 1)). It is interesting to note that the Minnesota experiment measured cardiac output by much more accurate methods. Using Roentgen kymographic volume measurements, these investigators found it to be reduced in the patient they describe to 44.8% of normal. Although the actual figures are different, this reduction is again in the range of the reduction described by the Warsaw investigators. Hence the conclusion reached in this study that minute volume or cardiac output is reduced was confirmed by Keys and co-workers and still stands today.

Since the pulse rate was found to be considerably lower than normal, the stroke volume was only slightly reduced (Figure 1). This reduction in stroke volume is 25% or less, whereas the reduction in cardiac output is often greater than 50%. Again the reduction in stroke volume described in the Minnesota experiment was of the same order of magnitude. The Minnesota group comments that with semistarvation the variability in measuring stroke volume doubles when compared to the same measurements before the semistarvation was imposed. No such data are available from the Warsaw ghetto study.

Electrocardiograms were taken of these patients and revealed regular but slow sinus rhythm, very low voltage, a normal ventricular system, low amplitude T waves, which were occasionally negative, and depressed ST segments. Moreover, on physical exertion there was very little change in the tracing. The authors conclude that the EKG findings suggest ischemia and "easy exhaustion" of the cardiac muscle. They further conclude that the fact that the EKG does not change after exertion indicates that the heart is functioning at the limit of its capability.

The most extensive EKG studies during semistarvation still remain those of Keys and co-workers. They describe their findings in great detail and devote an entire chapter of their book to the electrocardiogram. These studies, like the entire experiment, were truly remarkable and the reader is immediately struck by the detailed analysis which was undertaken in serial electrocardiograms taken during semistarvation and during recovery. The Minnesota group concludes that the most striking finding is the low amplitude of all peaks during the starvation period. They present a detailed discussion of the possible mechanisms for these findings and conclude that they represent changes within the heart muscle itself rather than extracardiac or positional factors. Thus their basic interpretation based on much more elegant data and much more detailed analysis is similar to that made by the Warsaw ghetto investigators. It is unfortunate that the actual tracings from the Warsaw study are not available; they would have been useful to the Minnesota group and to subsequent investigators. The one finding in the Warsaw study which is unique, since it was not studied by Keys and co-workers, was the lack of response to exercise. Again it is a great loss that the actual records were not recovered, since such recordings are almost nonexistent and since interpretation using modern techniques may have turned up subtle changes not noted by the Warsaw ghetto investigators.

From the studies so far described the authors conclude that the "dynamic reflexes end in hunger cachexia and the adaptive cardiac regulation becomes fixed . . . even at rest the heart is really in a stage of heart failure. . . ." Keys and his co-workers concluded after their studies ". . . the heart is certainly abnormal in starvation and does not maintain its circulatory function even in proportion to the reduced metabolic needs." Thus the concept of an adaptation at the expense of cardiac reserve was arrived at independently by both groups. Certainly the experience of many well meaning physicians who have thrown semistarved patients into cardiac failure as a result of too rapid refeeding bears out this interpretation.

Measurements of capillary circulation time and of oxygen consumption were made. The capillary circulation time was a method designed by the principal investigator to determine the time necessary for blood to circulate through the tissues fed by a particular artery and drained by a particular vein. Since the antecubital vessels were used, these were the tissues of the forearm and hand. This method obviously cannot measure circulation through any specific tissue, since the forearm and hand are made up of a variety of tissues. However, one might assume, and it would appear that the authors do, that this method can give some idea of the rate of blood flow through the muscle. In fact such procedures are being used in the "isolated perfusion techniques" employed by modern investigators attempting to study various metabolic events occurring in single organs or tissues. While absolute values probably are of little significance, the fact that in hunger disease the time necessary for the dye to appear in the vein is twice as long as in normal individuals is quite significant. Blood is circulating through the tissues more slowly. To my knowledge these were the first such observations ever made and I am not aware of subsequent studies that have examined this aspect of the circulatory difficulties in semistarvation.

Since the basal metabolic rate is reduced and the oxygen consumed per minute is reduced in hunger disease (see Tables 2 and 3), the authors suggest that this decrease in the rate of blood circulation through the tissues is a compensatory change which allows for more efficient oxygen utilization. The authors assume that there is reduced "tissue catabolism" and I must admit that I cannot see how they can reach that conclusion from these data. What I think they mean is that there is a decrease in overall metabolic rate in the various tissues. Certainly we cannot tell whether this is on the anabolic or the catabolic side. More recent data would suggest that at least certain catabolic events, for example, muscle protein breakdown, are much more rapid in semistarvation.

Investigators of the pressure within the vascular system at rest and after exercise in hunger disease complemented the findings of the hemodynamic observations. As had been previously reported, these investigators found reduced systolic and diastolic pressures and a low pulse pressure in hunger disease. What was perhaps more significant were their findings that exercise did not affect these pressures or their relationships (see Table 5 and Figure 2). Although previous studies and the subsequent Minnesota study had shown similar lowering of pressures at rest, none had examined the effect of exercise. Thus these investigators established for the first time not only systolic and diastolic hypotension but a "fixed hypotension" that could not respond to a normal physiological stimulus such as exercise.

Similar studies were carried out on venous pressure. Again, as had been previously noted, venous pressure tended to be low. Exercise had only a minimal effect on raising venous pressure.

Comparison of the results of the Warsaw study with the Minnesota study reveals certain differences. Although both studies demonstrated hypotension at rest in the arterial and the venous systems, the Minnesota volunteers had a slight lowering of arterial pressures and a much more marked lowering of venous pressure. The victims of the Warsaw ghetto starvation, by contrast, had a more marked lowering in arterial pressure, especially systolic pressure, and only a slight drop in venous pressure. The exact meaning of these differences is not totally clear but probably reflects the different nature and the different durations of the semistarvation in the two studies.

Based on the results which they obtained, the investigators draw certain conclusions and attempt to construct a pathophysiological picture of the dynamics of the circulatory system in hunger disease. They conclude that the adaptive response of the body in their patients was such as to "reduce the existence of their patients to a minimum." However, the adjustment is incomplete and is accompanied by certain pathologic changes. Blood volume increased and this was an unexpected finding and one which undoubtedly increased the strain on the heart. This increase was due to a tendency for water retention and a relative increase in the hydration of the plasma component. The volume of plasma increased from about 55% of total blood volume to about 70 to 75%. This results not only in hemodilution which, as we shall see, contributed to the anemia and leukopenia reported in the next chapter, but also in a reduction in the efficiency of the blood as a carrier of nutrients. Thus the vascular system is forced to supply more of this "poorly nourished" blood to the "hungry" tissues and organs. The absolute anemia (discussed in the next chapter) reduces the amount of oxygen carried by the blood and again increases the total blood requirements of the tissues even though they are consuming less oxygen. Thus there is an actual need for an increased volume of blood by the tissues. However, it is obvious that such an increase will place an increased demand on the heart. The authors note, however, that this increased demand rarely results in frank cardiac failure. They attribute this to other compensatory changes which tend to reduce cardiac work. For example, the slower circulation time decreases the cardiac work per minute and the reduced pulse rate allows the stroke volume to remain relatively normal. In addition, the authors speculate that the reduced capillary circulation time might allow for an increased time of exposure for nutrients and red cells to the tissues and hence might facilitate both nutrient and oxygen transfer. However, this "balance" is precarious at best since the system is unable to adapt further when placed under stress. In normal individuals, exertion increases tissue oxygenation and cardiac work. In hunger disease, there is little or no change; heart rate, stroke volume, systolic pressure, pulse pressure and EKGs remain the same.

Although no actual measurements of endocrine function were made, the investigators speculate on the possibility that endocrine involvement causes the circulatory effects they have observed. They cite the low BMR and lack of response to stress as a possible symptom of hypothyroidism or hypopituitarism. They note that cachexia and tissue atrophy are prominent symptoms of Simmonds' disease and that the pigmentation, hypotension, and hypothermia, as well as the low resistance to infection and the sexual changes, suggest adrenocortical dysfunction. Ovarian changes are suggested by the amenorrhea and parathyroid dysfunction by the bone changes. The only endocrine gland that shows no "obvious signs of dysfunction" is the pancreas.

The changes in the autonomic nervous system are described as a predominance of the parasympathetic over the sympathetic system. They note that this manifests itself during cardiovascular work by the slow pulse, the slow circulation time, the reduced arterial pressure, and the poor response to exercise.

The cardiovascular dysfunction caused by hunger disease, according to these investigators, constitutes a unique syndrome. Since only with difficulty can these "adaptive" changes sustain even basal metabolic levels, they consider that patients suffering from hunger disease are in a state of latent cardiac failure. However, they point out that the cardiovascular changes are quite different from those usually noted in cardiac insufficiency. There is no passive congestion of the peripheral organs or of the lungs, which on the contrary are relatively ischemic. They note that dyspnea and cyanosis are rare and that the edema is quite different from that seen in other types of cardiac failure. Even after exercise there was no increase in pulse rate or venous pressure. By contrast, there are certain similarities between the cardiovascular changes in hunger disease and in other types of cardiac dysfunction. In both, the slowing of the circulation is balanced by an increased blood volume and a diminished amount of work per minute of the heart. However, even here certain basic differences exist. In hunger disease, tissue oxygenation and basal metabolism are decreased; in other forms of cardiovascular dysfunction they are often increased.

This chapter, along with the previous one, represents the most sophisticated and the most difficult part of this remarkable study. The measurements made were suggested by careful clinical observation, and the best techniques available were used to make these measurements. The patients were carefully selected and the studies were carried out by a team of well trained and extremely careful investigators. The data obtained are sound and the variation due to intrinsic methodology is quite small. The pathophysiological changes inferred from these data are logical and certainly for the most part remain valid today. The interpretation of these changes was for the most part correct and has stood the test of time. Many of the findings have been subsequently confirmed. Some of the speculations are probably not correct, especially those involving the endocrine and perhaps the autonomic nervous systems. However, certainly they were logical and in addition they allow us even more insight into how these investigators thought. Obviously they were in tune with the latest theories and with the mainstream of research at that time. Although they were unable to substantiate some of their theories, they asked critical questions—questions which to this day have not been fully answered.

FIVE   Changes in Peripheral Blood and Bone Marrow in Hunger Disease

Dr. Michal Szejnman

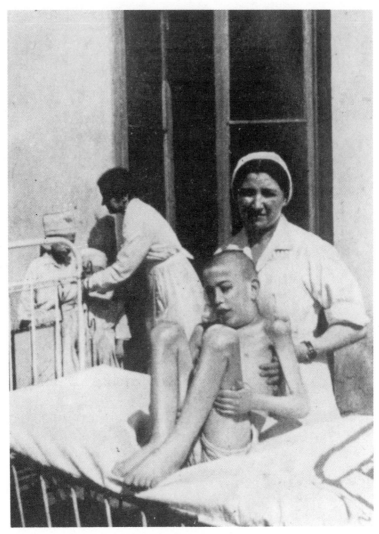

Ankylosis of the joints.

Several studies have established certain connections between the diet and the morphology of blood. Studies of scurvy started investigations into the relationship between vitamin deficiency and changes in blood. These studies established the lack of vitamin B_2 as the cause of pernicious anemia. By relating changes in the blood to vitamin deficiencies, blood pathology can be linked directly to the patient's nutrition. A diet inadequate in proteins or the inability to digest proteins can lead to serious liver disturbances such as sprue, or idiopathic steatorrhea. In these situations the pathogenesis is not clear, since we do not know if the findings are due to a lack of protein or to a lack of vitamin B. In the diseases just mentioned the diet was adequate in calories but of poor quality. By contrast, our patients consumed diets both low in calories and of poor quality. Although the literature concerned with the quality of the diet and blood morphology is very abundant, there have been only a few studies on the effect of quantitative hunger on blood morphology and there is general disagreement about the findings. Some authors deny the existence of hunger anemia; others believe there is an accompanying leukopenia and hypochromic anemia with anisocytosis of red cells. Autopsies have revealed bloody effusions, petechiae, and considerable increase in hemosiderin both microscopically and macroscopically. Bleeding diathesis was accompanied by anemia.

Some authors claim that these symptoms are caused by increased permeability of the capillaries, with serum and morphologic elements penetrating through the capillary walls into the tissues, causing edema, effusions, and anemia. Schlesinger, studying the relationship between neurological symptoms and anemia in hunger disease, emphasizes the frequent occurrence of a hyperchromic anemia that differs from pernicious anemia.

CLINICAL MATERIAL

Our research was of long duration. In our statistics we used data from patients with edema, dehydration, or slow heart action. We eliminated cases where we suspected complications or concomitant diseases. We considered only patients with no fever, no specific organ symptoms, negative results in tests for parasites and for blood in feces, lack of tuberculosis bacilli, and negative X-rays (this sometimes created a problem because we had to transport very sick people to a different building, and often did not have the facilities to do so. Therefore not all cases were X-rayed). Skin changes were considered very important. Our patients were mostly from refugee centers, where their living conditions were unsanitary. Almost all had lice, scabies, or pyoderma. The cases with extensive skin lesions were not included because of the possibilities of secondary eosinophilia and leukocytosis. Diagnostic difficulties were common also in cases with bloody diarrhea, because they often resembled dysentery. In spite of the negative results of serological and bacteriological examination taken at autopsy, purulent changes in the intestines looked very much like dysentery. We could not inoculate cultures for dysentery and therefore all of these cases were excluded from our statistics. However, blood tests were similar in all of the cases of acute diarrhea; that is, they showed extensive leukocytosis and some anemia, making them different from pure hunger disease.

Thus our study contained cases of true hunger disease, with edema, effusions in body cavities, and eventual dehydration, bradycardia, slight bloodless diarrhea, polyneuritis, and some changes similar to pellagra (one case). Our diagnosis was often confirmed at autopsy. If tuberculosis was found the case was excluded from our statistics.

In selecting cases for our study we used the following criteria:

1. Severe clinical symptoms.
2. Extensive edema.
3. Nervous system abnormalities.

4. Color of the skin. (In hunger disease it is pale as a result of edema, or pigmented as in Addison's disease. Sometimes the pallor is yellowish, like suntan. In these cases the blood abnormalities are most severe.)

We are not presenting our data in percentages but as actual number of cases. Only two people performed all the hematological determinations using the same equipment. Bone marrow was acquired with a needle and stained in the usual manner.

Red Blood Cells

Table 1 demonstrates that of 32 cases only six had 4 to 5 million red blood cells. Thus anemia was prevalent. The largest group of patients had 3 to 4 million red blood cells. Therefore we consider this number as average for slightly advanced hunger disease. Seven cases had only 2 to 3 million RBCs, seven cases only 1 to 2 million, and two cases below 1 million. The lowest red blood counts in the material we examined were 570,000 per cc and 670,000 per cc.

The color index was close to 1.0 (Table 2). In 10 cases it was 0.9, in eight cases it was 1.0. Lower color indices were rare (in one case 0.5 and in three cases 0.8). Indices of 1.1 were seen in seven cases, 1.2 in only three cases, and none were higher. Since most of the cases with a diminished number of RBCs had a color index of about 1, we can consider this a nor-

TABLE 1   RED BLOOD CELLS IN
HUNGER DISEASE

Red Blood Cells (millions)	Number of Cases
0–1	2
1–2	7
2–3	7
3–4	10
4–5	6
Above 5	0

TABLE 2   COLOR INDEX IN
HUNGER DISEASE

Amplitude of Color Index	Number of Cases
1.2	3
1.1	7
1.0	8
0.9	10
0.8	3
0.7	0
0.6	0
0.5	1

mochromic or, rarely, a hyperchromic anemia. Hypochromic anemia was very unusual. The value of the color index was independent of the number of RBCs. The two cases with the smallest number of RBCs had color indices of 0.9 and 1.2.

Summarizing all of the cases, we see that in the largest group, those with 3 to 4 million RBCs, the color index varied very little. The standard variation is ±0.2. In the group with 2 to 3 million red blood cells the standard variation is ±0.3 and in the group with 1 to 2 million red cells it is ±0.7 (Table 3). Most cases had a moderate reduction in the number of red cells and a color index around 1.0. In more advanced anemia the index shows greater variation. Sometimes it is reduced, but more often it is increased.

Examination of blood smears revealed anisocytosis without

TABLE 3   NUMBER OF RED BLOOD
CELLS AND COLOR INDEX

Red Blood Cells (millions)	Standard Variation of Color Index
0–1	0.3
1–2	0.7
2–3	0.3
3–4	0.2
4–5	0.2

Hunger Disease

TABLE 4   RETICULOCYTES AND PLATELETS IN
HUNGER CACHEXIA

Red Blood Cells (millions)	Reticulocytes (%)				Platelets (thousands)				
0–1	18								
1–2	12	15	31		63	98			
2–3	11	6	10	16	42	63	70	72	97	99
3–4	11	11	6	20		34	111			
4–5	11	7	8			117				

polychromasia or poikilocytosis. Anisocytosis was present in al-most every case regardless of the color index and the number of RBCs. In the same smear macrocytes, sometimes in large num-bers, appear next to microcytes. Intravital staining demon-strates a variable number of reticulocytes (Table 4).

In groups with 3 to 4 million or 4 to 5 million red cells there is occasionally a higher percentage of reticulocytes than normal, and often as anemia progresses the percentage increases up to 42%. By contrast, in some cases of anemia the number of retic-ulocytes was reduced and sometimes reticulocytes were com-pletely absent. Thus there is no relationship between the degree of anemia and the number of reticulocytes.

The osmotic resistance of the red blood cell is unchanged or perhaps slightly reduced. Hemolysis begins at around 0.54 (mostly 0.5) and ends from 0.26 to 0.42, usually around 0.32. For technical reasons we could not do the saponin test, which when positive is characteristic for pernicious anemia.

White Blood Cells

Like the red cells, the number of white blood cells was usually reduced. In eight cases, it was 4000 to 5000, in five cases 5000 to 6000, in three cases 6000 to 7000, and in two cases above 8000. Patients with bloody diarrhea, who are not included in these results, had a much more marked leukocytosis. The lowest white count in our study was 1100. A count of 2000 to 3000

TABLE 5   WHITE BLOOD CELLS
IN HUNGER DISEASE

White Blood Cells (thousands)	Number of Cases
0–1	0
1–2	1
2–3	4
3–4	5
4–5	8
5–6	5
6–7	1
7–8	3
Above 8	2

was found in four cases, and 3000 to 4000 in five cases (Table 5).

The differential smear was somewhat abnormal (Table 6). The percentage of neutrophils was slightly reduced and that of lymphocytes slightly increased. Six cases had advanced leukocytosis (70 to 80%), two cases had 50 to 60%, and one case 70 to 80% lymphocytes. The average percentage of leukocytes was 50 to 60% and of lymphocytes around 30%. There were few young forms in the peripheral blood except for cells with rod shaped nuclei. Two cases had 20%, one case 30%, and one case 40% of these cells. Eosinophils were seen only occasionally and there were few monocytes. Considering that the number of

TABLE 6   PERCENTAGE OF PARTICULAR CELL TYPES IN DIFFERENTIAL COUNT IN HUNGER DISEASE

Cell Type	Number of Cases										
	With 0%	With 0–10%	With 10–20%	With 20–30%	With 30–40%	With 40–50%	With 50–60%	With 60–70%	With 70–80%	With 80–90%	With 90–100%
Band forms	2	26	2	1	1						
Polymorphs			1	2	1	3	12	7	6		
Lymphocytes		2	4	10	9	4	2			1	
Monocytes	3	28	1								
Eosinophils	17	15									
Turck cells	27	5									

WBCs is diminished and the percentage of neutrophils is also reduced, we must conclude that the actual number of basophils is much lower than normal. If the lower limit of normal for basophils is 3500 to 4000, only three cases had a normal number, three cases were above normal, and 28 cases were below normal. The average number of basophils was 2500 to 3500; however, three cases had fewer basophils than 1000 per cc.

In only 10 cases were the number of lymphocytes lower than normal; in 17 cases lymphocyte number was increased, and in seven cases there were normal numbers of lymphocytes (Table 7).

White blood cells in smears sometimes showed pathological granulations. Among the lymphocytes there are many young forms; some even have nucleoli in the nuclei. However these cannot be considered lymphoblasts because of the appearance of the cytoplasm.

There was no relation between red blood cell and white blood cell counts. On the average, the numbers of RBCs and WBCs were diminished, but more advanced anemia is not paralleled by advanced leukopenia, nor is the reverse true. One case had 670,000 RBCs and 5000 WBCs, another case had 2,400,000 RBCs and only 1000 WBCs.

TABLE 7   POLYMORPHS AND LYMPHOCYTES IN HUNGER DISEASE

Number of Leukocytes (thousands)	Polymorphs (Number of Cases)	Lymphocytes (Number of Cases)
0–0.5	0	3
0.5–1	3	7
1 –1.5	6	7
1.5–2.0	7	9
2.0–2.5	2	5
2.5–3.0	5	2
3.0–3.5	5	1
3.5–4.0	3	0
4.0–4.5	2	0
4.5–5.0	1	0
Above 5.0	0	0

Studying blood morphology in "pure" hunger disease helps in interpreting the blood morphology when hunger is complicated by other diseases, such as petechial typhus. In the second year of the epidemic of typhus, unlike the first year, there was often leukopenia with relative lymphocytosis and the absence of eosinophils. Some monocytes and Turck cells were present. The leukopenia and lymphocytosis could be the result of hunger disease, while the monocytosis and the presence of Turck cells are specific for typhus.

Blood Platelets

The number of platelets is reduced, from 65,000 to 34,000 (Table 4). There is no relationship among the number of RBCs, WBCs, and platelets. There is no bleeding diathesis in spite of the low platelet count. In 2 years we did not see one case of bleeding diathesis in our hospital. Observations from other hospitals and refugee centers confirm the rarity of bleeding diathesis in contrast to the situation during World War I, when bleeding diathesis was one of the classic features of semistarvation.

Bone Marrow

In nine patients we were able to study the bone marrow (Table 8). In two cases we had to puncture the sternum twice and in one case we had to puncture the sternum three times in different spots and were still unable to obtain marrow. In this case the marrow had become fibrous and devoid of cells. This finding was not expected from the blood morphology. In one case the second examination revealed a much richer bone marrow than at the first examination, although the patient's general condition and peripheral blood morphology were much worse. In all cases of hunger disease the barrier between bone marrow and peripheral blood is probably enhanced.

In those cases in which the bone marrow was rich in cells only once did we observe a shift toward young forms. In this case these were mostly myelocytes with normal numbers of my-

TABLE 8 BONE MARROW IN HUNGER DISEASE

Bone Marrow	Cases										Number of Cases
	1	2	3	4	5	6	7	8	9	10	
Cellular elements											
Many	+		+	+					+	+	5
Few					±		±	±			3
None		−				−					2
Shift to the left											
Large	+		+	+				+	+	+	6
Slight					±		±				2
None		−				−					2
Lymphocytosis											
Severe		+				+		+			3
Mild					±		±				2
None	−		−	−					−	−	5
Ratio of white blood cells to red blood cells	1.3	4	2.4	4	6	4	2.1	1.1	1	2.7	

eloblasts and promyelocytes. We did not observe any giant cells as described by Tempka and Brown in pernicious anemia. In those bone marrows that were poor in cells, lymphocytes were prevalent. In most cases there was a shift from WBC production toward RBC production. The shift involved normoblasts and not the youngest forms. We did not observe true megaloblastic RBCs, and only once were there atypical young RBCs resembling megaloblasts. Macrocytosis was as obvious in the bone marrow as in the peripheral blood.

From the material presented above we can visualize the usual blood morphology in hunger disease. We did not find any relationship between the clinical symptoms and the blood picture. Very severe clinical symptoms could be accompanied by mild anemia and, conversely, severe anemia or leukopenia might accompany mild hunger disease. We have no explanation for this lack of correlation. Some patients were dried out completely, with rigid wrinkled skin, hoarse voices, due probably to dried out laryngeal mucosa, color indices around 1.0, and numerous RBCs.

The small number of WBCs in some cases and the increased

number in others excludes the increased blood density as an explanation of the increase in RBCs. Several times we were able to examine blood a few hours before death. The blood picture was normal and no drastic changes were observed. On the contrary, the peripheral blood was quite active, with large numbers of reticulocytes.

In some patients with very low WBC counts we might have expected clinical symptoms of granulocytopenia and agranulocytosis. However, there were no abscesses in the throat, there was no strep throat, and infectious processes were not more severe than in patients without hunger disease. Patients with infection sometimes had a mild leukocytosis, but sometimes there was no reaction. One patient before and during the formation of a large abscess on his palm had a persistent WBC count of 4000. Another patient, in spite of a tremendous abscess of the calf, had a WBC count of 2400. In one boy the WBC count increased from 7200 to 8200 and in one woman from 2800 to 7800 during periods of active infection.

The mode of reacting to infection was therefore dependent not on the general clinical state of the patient but on the ability of the bone marrow to respond. We tried to find an explanation for the lack of correlation between changes in the blood and the general state of the patient.

With this purpose in mind, we examined the blood of people suffering from hunger for a very long time but without clinical symptoms of hunger disease. The changes described above were also present in this population. White blood cell counts were often reduced to 4000, with only 40% neutrophils. Red blood cell counts were around 2.5 to 3 million, and almost every smear showed anisocytosis and macrocytosis. These changes caused us to reevaluate our clinical reliance on blood morphology. Before the war if we observed these changes in red and white blood cells we would suspect a blood disease and often decide on a transfusion. Today we know that these people are able to work and have no symptoms of any disease. For example, we observed two sisters who spent the war years together, both consuming the same very poor diet. One of them lost 30% of her original body weight, and her blood picture showed all the symptoms of hunger disease. The other maintained her weight and had a completely normal blood picture. Therefore, we examined a group of individuals who were eating relatively well, qualitatively and quantitatively, and who for various reasons were losing weight. Although these cases were never hungry, they still usually showed the same changes in blood morphology. We concluded that the changes in blood were not the result of caloric or qualitative undernutrition but were the result of physicochemical changes due to weight loss.

In spite of the overall lack of correlation between the clinical symptoms and the blood picture, there are some cases where the relationship is very close (Table 9, Case a). The worsening of clinical symptoms was followed by advancing leukopenia and anemia with an increasing color index. The story of Case b in Table 9 is very interesting in this regard. The patient had severe polyneuritis, but when her clinical symptoms started improving, when she started to walk again, and her edema disappeared, her WBC count and also the morphology of the white cells improved considerably.

In some cases the changes in blood overshadow the patient's clinical state, making one wonder whether the blood changes are accompanying the hunger disease or whether hunger disease is the result of existing bone marrow disease. However, careful analysis of our material proves without doubt that quantitative and qualitative undernutrition is the basis of both the clinical and the hematological findings.

DISCUSSION OF THE CASES

Case 1. Patient B came to the hospital because of diarrhea, edema, and limited mobility. He was experiencing progressive weakness and akwardness and could not perform such simple tasks as fastening a button. He stopped walking, the edema in his lower extremities and abdomen increased considerably, and he complained of a burning sensation in the tongue, and diar-

TABLE 9 SUMMARY OF FINDINGS IN PERIPHERAL BLOOD

Case Number	Date	Hb	Number of White Blood Cells	Number of Red Blood Cells (millions)	Color Index	Reticulocytes (%)	Platelets	White Blood Cells						Remarks
								Segmented Neutrophils	Band-formed Neutrophils	Lymphocytes	Monocytes	Eosinophils	Turck Cells	
a	April 30	81	9200	4.5	0.9	—	—	34.5	26.5	37	2	0	0	—
	May 19	55	4000	2.8	1.0	—	—	53	34	10	3	0	0	—
b	June 7	76.5	3400	3.3	1.1	—	—	17	3	78	1	1	0	Anisocytosis
	August 6	72	4900	3.2	1.1	—	—	56.5	5.5	36.5	0	1.5	0	Slight aniso-cytosis
1	March 23	50	5200	2.0	1.2	12	—	30	8	57	5	0	0	Anisocytosis
	May 11	51	3300	2.5	1.02	4	—	76	3	14	5	2	0	Rx–Fe, HCl
	May 21	56	2200	2.7	1.03	6	73,000	62	6	29	2	1	0	Rx, Fe, HCl
	June 1	65	3100	3.0	1.08	2	75,000	59	3	34	2	2	0	Rx, Fe, HCl
3	March 26	55	2400	2.4	1.1	1	—	76	4	16	4	0	0	Anisocytosis, macrocytosis
	April 11	70	3500	3.3	1.06	1	—	57	13	22	5	1	2	Rx, Fe, Zymaze
	June 9	56	1000	2.4	1.16	1	38,000	54	6	34	6	0	0	Rx–Blood in salad
4	March 31	31	3900	1.7	0.9	—	—	50	3	44	1	1	1	Anisocytosis, macrocytosis
5	April 25	48	2200	2.1	1.1	3	—	44	6	40	5	5	0	Rx, Fe
	February 28	11	5400	0.7	0.9	18	—	77.0	2	16	5	0	0	Anisocytosis, oligochromic
	March 23	21	2400	1.1	0.9	18	—	68	0	30	1	1	0	Rx–Fe
	April 13	52	2900	2.8	0.8	—	—	49	2	35	13	1	1	Rx transfusion

rhea. There was no blood or mucus in the feces. The history of undernutrition dated back to the outbreak of the war.

Physical examination revealed far advanced cachexia, brown pigmentation in various areas of the skin, with other areas appearing white with a yellowish tinge, advanced edema of the lower extremities, lower back, and abdomen, muscular atrophy of the forearms and hands, and some free fluid in the pleural and abdominal cavities.

Laboratory examination showed normal urine and feces and reduced gastric content. The blood morphology is shown in Table 9, Case 1. Neurological examination confirmed the diagnosis of polyneuritis. We attempted to obtain bone marrow prior to initiating liver therapy. However, out of 120 cases this was the only one where in spite of several trials we could not obtain any marrow. We concluded that the marrow was replaced by fibrous tissue. For technical reasons it was impossible to X-ray the patient. Therapy with liver resulted in no improvement. A trial of iron and hydrochloric acid was also unsuccessful. Combined HCl, iron, and sykoton improved the blood count and lowered the color index. The leukocyte count changed very little. Clinically the patient improved after a better diet and after the administration of Betabion and strychnine. Dehydration by inducing acidosis and by administering mercurial diuretics did not affect either the blood or the patient's general state. The leukopenia persisted and the reticulocyte count dropped shortly before the patient died. Observations during the last few days of life and post mortem examination were impossible because of the deportation. The diagnosis in this case was uncertain—either pernicious anemia or hunger anemia. Since liver therapy was ineffective and there was no urobilinogen increase in urine even with the characteristic neurological symptoms, we decided upon hunger with edema and cachexia and excluded pernicious anemia. The blood morphology was not helpful because in pernicious anemia megaloblasts are not always present in the smear, and the lack of HCl was also not diagnostic. However, there are known cases of pernicious anemia with concomitant polyneuritis without other types of changes.

Case 2. Patient Z was transferred from the neurological department. The patient came in because of loss of sensation and movement in the lower extremities and attacks of shaking tremor. A diagnosis of polyneuritis and spasmophilia was made. There was no change in the RBC count, although the WBC count came down to 2700. As the general condition of the patient deteriorated a rapid progressive anemia developed, with a color index of 1.0. In addition there was a lack of gastric juice and a burning sensation in the mouth. The bone marrow had some promegaloblasts. However, we did not believe this to be pernicious anemia. We diagnosed it as a case of hunger disease, but the blood morphology was not characteristic enough to support our diagnosis. Examination of the bone marrow is seen in Table 10, Case 2. There were no giant rod shaped bodies in the white cells as described by Tempka and Brown. There were a number of atypical red blood cells, but no promegaloblasts or megaloblasts. There were discrepancies in the maturity of the cytoplasm and the nuclei, many amitoses, and cells with two nuclei. Very few mitoses were seen and different types of normoblasts prevailed over younger forms (proerythroblasts). With this type of red cell morphology even if some cells look like megaloblasts the diagnosis of pernicious anemia is not appropriate. We believe that in this case there was severe damage to the bone marrow, which first affected the WBCs and later the RBCs. Since the urobilinogen in urine was not increased, indicating no increased destruction of RBCs, a typical symptom of pernicious anemia, we assumed that hunger anemia had changed into aplastic anemia. The further course of the disease confirmed our hypothesis. We could not prove the diagnosis of aplastic anemia, but the patient did not improve after large doses of Campolon and fresh raw liver administered in salad. The general state of the patient improved after the first transfusion but the blood picture did not change. After a lapse of time the patient developed effusions in the left pleural space and after a second transfusion the patient died. Autopsy did not disclose the characteristic changes of pernicious anemia in the gastric mu-

TABLE 10 BONE MARROW

Types of Cell	Percent of Total Cells			
	Case 2	Case 3	Case 4	Case 5
Erythroblasts				
Proerythroblasts	0.6	0	0.8	0.4 0.5 0.8
Erythroblasts	0.4	0.4	3.0	2.2 0.4 1.6
Basophils	4.2	2.8	9.6	22.4 7.2 21.4
Normoblasts				
Polychromatophils	1.2	5	6.6	6.4 8.8 7.4
Orthochromatophils	5.4	4	4.4	5.6 9.2 6.6
Promegaloblasts	0			
Nontypical	2.6	0	0.8	
Mitosis	0			
Amitosis, 2 nuclei cells	2.4	0	0.4	
Leukoblasts				
Myeloblasts	0.6	0.4	0.2	0 0 0
Promyelocytes	2.2	0.8	1.8	1 3 0.6
Myelocytes				
Neutrophils	32.2	6.8	16.4	16.4 6.4 5.8
Eosinophils	2.6	0.8	0.6	2 0.4 0
Metamyelocytes				
Neutrophils	10.0	9.4	19.2	9.2 4.6 13.0
Eosinophils	0	0	0	0 0 0
Band forms				
Neutrophils	1.4	6	16.6	5.8 12.4 13.4
Eosinophils	0	0	0	0 0 0
Polymorphs				
Neutrophils	6.6	2.3	4.4	13.4 25.4 7.0
Eosinophils	2.2	0.4	0.2	1 2.0 0.2
Basophils	0.2	20	0	
Reticuloendothelials				
R-cells				
Macrophages	0.6	0	0.2	0 0.2 0
Lymphocytes	0	0	0	0 0 0
Plasma cells	1.6	0.6	2.2	2 1.4 0.4
Mesenchymal	0	0	0	0 0.2 0
Lymphocytes	10.0	36.6	11.8	8.4 15.8 21
Monocytes including	2.0	2.4	0.4	1.8 1.4 0.8
nondifferentiated	2.0	0	0.6	0
leukocytes				
Erythrocytes	4	4	2.4	1.3 1.1 1.1

cosa and the tongue. Macroscopic examination did not disclose any deposition of hemosiderin.

Case 3 (see Tables 9 and 10). This patient came to the hospital from a labor camp because of general weakness and edema. Examination showed cachexia, and edema of the face, lumbar parts, and extremities. There was no ascites. The pulse rate was 48 and irregular. While in the hospital the patient developed effusions in both pleural cavities and in the abdominal cavity. An abscess on his palm healed without complications. During one remission he left the hospital but came back after a few days in poor condition. Neurological examination was normal. The digestive system was normal except for occasional diarrhea after oral administration of the iron preparations. The urine, feces, and stomach contents were normal. Upon admission to the hospital, blood study revealed advanced anemia with hyperchromia and macrocytosis, a leukopenia with normal WBC morphology, and a very low reticulocyte count (0 to 1 per thousand). Bone marrow was very poor, with a predominance of lymphocytes. In the red cell system there were macrocytes among normoblasts and normocytes, but the quantitative relationship was normal. The bone marrow had almost no reticulocytes, a very bad prognostic sign. Therapy with Zymaris, Betabion, and iron transiently increased the RBC count and hemoglobin and decreased the color index. However the reticulocyte count remained very low. The general condition of the patient became much worse, with concomitant worsening of the blood morphology. Hemoglobin and RBC count continued to drop, anisocytosis with giant macrocytes appeared, WBC count was 1000, and platelet count was only 38,400. Sternal bone marrow was rich in cells, showing mild stimulation of the erythroblastic system without evidence of pathological forms. There was a leukocytosis with a shift toward myelocytes. Very few platelets and megakaryocytes were seen, and only 1 per 1000 reticulocytes could be counted. After transfusion the patient did not improve; he developed fever for the first time, and died. The transfusion did not change his blood findings. Aside from all the findings of hunger disease, autopsy revealed fresh tubercles on the right pleura. The liquid effusion in all the cavities was lymphatic and there were no changes in the chest cavity glands or in the lungs. We believed that the shock of the transfusion triggered an exacerbation of a tuberculosis infection, causing the fever and the fresh foci in the lungs.

The diagnosis in this case is aplastic anemia because of continuous diminution in blood elements and the absence of signs of regeneration. The abundance of cells in the bone marrow demonstrates that their release was completely inhibited; the barrier between marrow and periphery became very strong and the various morphological elements would not reach the circulating blood. The reason for this block in release is unknown. Schulten in his monograph on bone marrow mentions the possibility of anemia with either very rich or very poor bone marrow.

Case 4 (see Tables 9 and 10). This patient's clinical history was characteristic for hunger disease. The patient had advanced anemia, color index 0.1, and leukopenia with relative lymphocytosis. The smear showed anisocytosis with a preponderance of macrocytes. Oral and intravenous iron therapy improved the blood count and hemoglobin and the color index rose. When iron therapy was stopped the RBC count diminished slightly but never went back to the original low levels. The color index decreased to 0.8, the WBC count decreased, and the reticulocyte count was normal. Bone marrow was rich in cells of the red cell series, and there was a shift to the left in the white cell series toward myelocytes without pathological forms. Since clinically the patient improved markedly, even more than his blood picture, he was discharged.

Case 5 (see Tables 9 and 10). This patient came to the hospital because of profound weakness and edema. Previously he had suffered from diarrhea and a burning tongue. His nutrition was very poor. His color was strikingly pale with a yellow hue. He had edema of the feet and lumbar parts. The patient walked with difficulty. Examination of urine, feces, and stomach contents detected diminished HCl. Blood tests showed 670,000 RBC per cc with anisocytosis, reticulocytosis (18 per 1000 reticulocytes), and leukopenia with normal morphology. Bone marrow was moderately rich in cells, with some stimulation of erythroblasts and a slight shift to the left of leukoblasts. None of these symptoms is specific for any definite hematological entity. The laboratory tests excluded pernicious anemia, hypochromic anemia, or chlorosis. We could exclude hemorrhage or loss of blood by destruction and therefore we diagnosed our case as hunger anemia.

As for therapy, we tried to improve the patient's diet. We gave him Zymase which improved his RBC count, color index, and reticulocytes, but the leukopenia became worse. Iron therapy did not help and therefore the patient received 120 cc of blood, which helped at once. The WBC count rose to 7300 and then fell back to 2700 because of post-transfusion bone marrow inhibition, and finally started to improve slowly but continuously while maintaining the same hemoglobin and RBC count. Bone marrow did not show any changes. Clinically the patient improved as much as his blood picture, and was discharged to return for follow up, but the deportations had just started and we never saw him again. During his three months in the hospital with repeated laboratory examinations the only reason found for the anemia was hunger. This diagnosis was confirmed by the fact that an adequate diet was more efficient than medication in fighting the anemia.

PATHOGENESIS OF BLOOD CHANGES IN HUNGER

After presenting the results of our study and some of the more interesting cases we would like to discuss the pathogenesis of the blood changes in hunger. The alterations in water metabolism necessitate considering the circulating elements in the periphery. We examined the volume of circulating blood and the hematocrit index. The study demonstrated that in people with edema as well as in those with dry cachexia the volume of blood was diminished less than the weight. Thus there was an increased blood volume per kilogram of body weight. The hematocrit index was also lowered; therefore, in hunger there is dilution of blood. We do not know whether hunger anemia originates because of hypofunction of the bone marrow, because of improper marrow release, or because of increased blood volume. If this last reason is valid, we must consider hunger anemia hypervolemic oligocytemic, according to the latest classification.

It has been shown many times that macrocytosis could be of peripheral origin. In serious disturbances of water metabolism, as occur in hunger disease, there are changes in osmotic pressure and concomitant swelling of red cells. In favor of this concept is the fact that the macrocytosis occurred in patients with a color index equal to or even less than 1.0. In addition the fact that a strong correlation between anemia and weight loss occurred in nonhungry patients added weight to the circulatory explanation.

By contrast in a few cases, after suitable acidification, we gave a diuretic and some patients lost as much as 5 liters of fluid with no change in blood morphology. This demonstrates a lack of correlation between water metabolism and the blood picture. As we mentioned before, changes in RBCs, WBCs, and platelets do not occur in parallel. Dilution of blood would be expected to have the same effect on all three systems. A patient might have severe leukopenia and normal RBCs or just the opposite. Also the same patient might have changing WBCs with stable RBCs. The anemia can be improving and WBC count dropping. These results definitely exclude blood dilution as the only reason for the anemia. The changes in blood morphology exclude peripheral blood as the only factor. We demonstrated that the number of lymphocytes as a rule does not diminish whereas the number of granulocytes drops precipitously. Again we cannot assume that only leukocytes undergo dilution.

Macrocytosis could also be of peripheral origin, but in our cases it was concomitant with increased color index. Therefore it was connected with increased amounts of hemoglobin in the RBCs. In idiopathic hypochromic anemia there are macrocytes and a low color index, which demonstrates that not every macrocytosis with a low color index is of peripheral origin. Besides in our cases there were always not only macrocytes but also microcytes present, and it would be difficult to conceive of the same physicochemical factor as responsible for bloating and shrinkage of red cells.

Macrocytosis was present not only in the circulating blood but also in the bone marrow. In most of our cases the bone marrow was rich in cells, the increased number of reticulocytes resulting from stimulation of erythroblasts, demonstrating that certain changes originate during blood formation.

The appearance of symptoms of hunger disease in people who were not hungry but lost weight is consistent with our thesis. If the diet was adequate, these people would not be losing 20 to 30% of their weight. The large weight loss indicates increased individual caloric needs or abnormalities in the absorbing process. Both qualitative and quantitative hunger can appear when absorption or assimilation is defective. Under these conditions the symptoms of hunger disease appear in spite of good nutrition and the changes in blood are the same as in cases of malnutrition.

This discussion makes clear the fact that the increase in circulating water can aggravate existing anemia, but it cannot be its only cause. For the real cause we must look elsewhere.

THERAPY

Since hunger is the cause of the blood changes, we tried the following modes of therapy, the results of which are shown in Table 11.

Raw Animal Blood in Food

We added raw animal blood to food in a salad. Although we hoped this would improve the hematologic state, in all cases results were negative. In spite of the salad, the anemia progressed. Analysis of the feces showed a positive benzidine reaction, indicating a disturbance in the process of absorption.

TABLE 11   RESULTS OF THERAPY

Therapy Used	Number of Cases	Hb	Color Index	Red Blood Cells	White Blood Cells	General Results
Blood salad	5	—	—	—	—	—
Fe	6	+	+	+	Irrit.	—
Liver	2	—				—
Liver, Fe, HCl	1	+	+	+	±	±
Zymase B'	2	—				—
Transfusion	3	+	+	+	+	Positive 1 Negative 2
Diet	2	±	+	+	+	+

Intravenous Iron

Since oral iron therapy was not recommended because of its laxative effect, we tried to give the patients intravenous injections of iron. The side effects were numerous: malaise, accelerated heart beat, hot flushes, and sweating. Locally the injections were painful; the vein would become hard and no longer suitable for injections. Only two patients received the full course of six injections each; the others received only three or four. The effect of iron, regardless of the method of administration, was fleeting and insignificant. Hemoglobin and color index would rise transiently, often without any change in the blood count. In one case normochromic anemia changed into hyperchromic. After iron therapy was stopped the situation reverted back.

Liver Therapy

Two cases received liver therapy without effects. Hunger anemia cannot be classified in the category of pernicious anemia. The bone marrow morphology is completely different in spite of the similarities in the peripheral blood. The pathogenesis is also different in these two types of anemia. In pernicious anemia, because of the lack of a specific intrinsic factor, red cells are abnormal, are less resistent, and disintegrate prematurely. The increased hemolysis increases the quantity of urobilinogen in urine and hemosiderin deposits in tissues. The bone marrow, in an attempt to compensate for the hemolyzing cells, undergoes hypertrophy and therefore at autopsy we find deep red marrow. One might assume that in hunger there would be complicating factors, such as scurvy, steatorrhea, or celiac disease, which could result in symptoms similar to those in pernicious anemia. But it is not so. In hunger disease the red blood cells do not hemolyze abnormally rapidly, urobilinogen in the urine is not increased, and at autopsy macroscopic examination does not reveal hemosiderin in the tissues. Instead there is inadequate formation of red blood cells or inadequate movement from the marrow to the peripheral blood. We must emphasize that the differential diagnosis between pernicious anemia and hunger anemia is possible only after bone marrow examination and the results of a trial of liver therapy. Clinical symptoms like the lack of urobilinogen in the urine or nervous system abnormalities are not sufficient. During World War I, from 1914 through 1918, when bone marrow examination and liver therapy were not known, many cases of pernicious anemia were described. Those were probably cases of hyperchromic macrocytic hunger anemia and not pernicious anemia.

Combined Iron and Liver Therapy

Since iron and liver therapy were ineffective we decided to combine them (as recommended by Tempka). This author described many cases of pernicious anemia, especially hypochromic pernicious anemia, with good therapeutic results from combined iron and liver therapy. We had some improvement in one case and this was not as complete as that described by Tempka.

Vitamin Therapy

We tried to consider hunger disease as an avitaminosis, since we knew from the literature that lack of vitamin B_2 can produce hyperchromic anemia, although the exact relationship between B_2 and the anemia is not completely clear. We tried to give our patients an extract of yeast containing B complex. In two cases the results were negative. This was not surprising because the ghetto diet contained vitamin B (black bread, oats, kasha). Avitaminosis B_1, pellagra, and avitaminosis C, scurvy, were practically nonexistent. Generally speaking, in the ghetto, in spite of the lack of vitamins in the food, there were no symptoms of pure avitaminosis, such as rickets, night blindness, or dryness of the conjunctiva.

Small Transfusions

Small transfusions (120 to 200 cc) worked poorly. In one case transfusion resulted in aggravation of symptoms and death. In a second case there was transitory general improvement while in the third case the improvement was stable but the transfusion was not the only therapeutic measure employed.

Food

The best results were achieved by supplying adequate nutrition and food with an appropriate caloric value. These results could be anticipated because the only rational therapy for hunger is food.

CONCLUSIONS

1. Prolonged hunger results in a reduction in all morphologic elements in blood and an increase in the percentage of reticulocytes (Tables 1 through 4).

2. Anemia is normochromic or hyperchromic and only very rarely hypochromic. There is anisocytosis with a predominance of macrocytes.

3. Granulocytes are more deficient than lymphocytes (Table 6).

4. There is no correlation between changes in RBCs and WBCs, blood morphology, and the clinical state of the patient.

5. Bone marrow is more active in producing cells than in releasing them into peripheral blood. Therefore the bone marrow is very rich in cells.

6. In some cases the bone marrow retains the ability to react to stimuli with leukocytosis; in more advanced stages it becomes "rigid" or results in aplastic anemia.

7. The cause of anemia is not increased RBC destruction or increased volume of circulating water.

8. Since the anemia is the result of a lack of all kinds of food, proper diet is the only therapy.

9. No clinical or hematological symptoms connected with avitaminosis were observed.

10. The patient's general condition and to a lesser extent the ability of his bone marrow to respond play a role in the anemia.

Epicrisis of Case 2

Rich bone marrow; anisocytosis with prevalent macrocytes. Very few mitoses and platelets. Numerous destroyed cells. Abnormal marrow containing atypical cells; chromatophilic normoblasts with basophilic granules. Many amitotic cells with two nuclei.

Epicrisis of Case 3

1. Bone marrow poor in cells. Numerous platelets, no mitoses, very few isolated nuclei or degenerating cells. Considerable anisocytosis, macrocytosis among normocytes and normoblasts. Turck cells with two nuclei. Many large young lymphocytes, some with nucleoli.
2. Bone marrow moderately rich in cells. No mitoses, very few platelets, many destroyed white blood cells. Anisocytosis less intensive than in the peripheral blood.

Epicrisis of Case 4

Rich bone marrow, full of cells. Numerous platelets, no mitosis, no degenerating cells, antisocytosis, mild macrocytosis.

Epicrisis of Case 5

1. At the beginning of clinical observations, bone marrow with few cells; some netlike degenerating cells. In the leukoblasts a shift to the left. Stimulation of the erythroblast series.
2. Just before transfusion, bone marrow with few cells; no cell division. A few degenerating cells and isolated nuclei. Very few platelets, many atypical lymphocytes. Anisocytosis and macrocytosis of the red cells.

EDITOR'S COMMENTS

Myron Winick, M.D.

This chapter represents an attempt to describe the changes in peripheral blood and bone marrow in the patients suffering from hunger disease. These studies were quantitative and employed well established techniques that were in use at the time. However, there is another facet of these investigations that not only gives us some clues to the nature of the hematological deficiencies in these patients but also gives us a good deal of insight into the characters of the physicians carrying out the study. A number of different therapeutic interventions were introduced and the responses to the therapy were noted. None was successful, and hence certain causes for the anemia or leukopenia could be ruled out. One gets the feeling, however, that the investigators were concerned with more than generating data. They were looking for a way to "cure" the hematologic deficit which might benefit those suffering from hunger disease. They concluded out of frustration that specific therapy is of little use and that only supplying an adequate diet will restore the hematologic status to normal.

At the beginning of the chapter the distinction between hematologic findings secondary to qualitative malnutrition, that is, deficiency of a single nutrient, and quantitative malnutrition as seen in hunger disease, is clearly pointed out. The bleeding seen in scurvy and the changes in pernicious anemia are cited as deficiencies of single nutrients. It is interesting that this is pointed out before the identification of vitamin B_{12}. They note that in quantitative undernutrition there is little agreement about the hematologic findings. An attempt was made therefore to limit the cases studied to those with "pure" hunger disease. Patients with infections were excluded from the study as were those suffering from any complicating disease.

Most of their patients had a normochromic anemia. Both microcytes and macrocytes were present and the blood smears showed both anisocytosis and poikilocytosis. Some patients had many reticulocytes and others none in their peripheral smears. Osmotic fragility was normal in most of the cases studied. The extent of the anemia varied from severe to moderate. Thus, with respect to the red blood cell picture, results were quite variable. In addition, the severity of anemia bore no relation either to the type of anemia or to the number of reticulocytes seen. This heterogeneity of response has been noted many times both before and since this study was performed. For example, anemia may or may not occur in children suffering from severe nutritional marasmus. Children with frank kwashiorkor often show only a mild or moderate anemia similar in quality to the anemia described in this chapter. Many studies before and during World War I report moderate to severe anemia in persons suffering from hunger and inadequate nutrition. In the Minnesota study the changes in red blood cells could be observed serially in the same patient. The average hemoglobin was 13 g at the start of the experiment and dropped to around 11.8 g by the end of the starvation period. Red blood cell count dropped from 5.2 million to 3.8 million, color index remained around 1, and hematocrit dropped from 46.8 to 36.4%. Thus, the anemia was moderate in degree and normochromic and slightly macrocytic in type, essentially the same findings as reported in this study. It is interesting to note that the drop in hemoglobin during the first half of the starvation period in the Minnesota study was much greater (2.5 g) than in the second half of the starvation period (0.9 g). This suggests that the anemia tends to develop rapidly and then to reach a plateau. The very low hemoglobin levels and red cell counts described in this chapter in a few of the patients and the reports in the literature of equally low values after prolonged starvation suggest that in at least certain patients, after very long starvation a further breakdown occurs in the organism's ability to maintain relatively stable red cell indices. The anemia in these cases becomes progressively worse and may contribute to the patients' ultimate demise.

Before the studies reported in this chapter were undertaken the literature describing the changes in white blood cells during long term starvation showed very little consistency. While the majority of reports indicated a leukopenia, some noted no changes in white cell number and a few described leukocytosis. This study confirms the majority of previous observations and demonstrates a moderate to severe leukopenia. In addition, the proportion of lymphocytes was increased to about 30% of the total number of white blood cells. Many of the lymphocytes were described as young cells, some even containing nucleoli; however, none were considered to be lymphoblasts. No relation was found between the number of red blood cells and the number of white blood cells for any given patient. The response to an infection such as typhus called forth monocytes and Turck cells which appeared in the peripheral blood, but the leukopenia and relative lymphocytosis persisted. An interesting observation made in this study was the virtual absence of eosinophils, even with certain infections. This may be part of the overall decreased allergic response that was noted in these patients. However, it should be pointed out that in studies made in American prisoners released from Japanese prison camps after World War II, marked eosinophilia was reported in many patients. Assuming that the eosinophilia was due to superimposed malaria or other parasitic diseases, this finding suggests that under certain conditions an eosinophilic response can be called forth.

The Minnesota study essentially confirmed what was found by the Warsaw investigators. Leukopenia was again noted, but the proportion of lymphocytes remained normal. These investigators note that the increased blood volume which would result in a relative leukopenia was not enough to account for the degree of leukopenia in the Minnesota volunteers. Exactly the same observation was made by the Warsaw investigators in trying to explain the anemia and leukopenia that they observed. The Minnesota experiment, of course, could quantitate the degree of leukopenia by comparing prestarvation levels to levels at the end of the starvation period in the same individuals. The results indicate a drop of 24.1% after correction for the increased plasma volume. During rehabilitation, there was significant recovery of the leukocyte count which was again not explainable by the small decrease in blood volume that occurred during this period. The investigators explain this increase as either a relative increase in production over destruction of white cells during rehabilitation or a release of white cells which had been sequestered in organs and tissues during the starvation period.

Platelet counts were reduced from 65,000 to about 34,000 in the Warsaw patients. In spite of this, however, there was no bleeding diathesis noted either in the patients actually studied or in observations made in other hospitals or in refugee centers. This was in marked contrast to what had occurred during World War I, when bleeding diathesis was a very prominent feature of semistarvation. Although platelet counts in peripheral blood were not done in the Minnesota experiment, no bleeding was reported in any of the patients. The data from Warsaw and from Minnesota, as well as from a number of subsequent observations, suggest that spontaneous bleeding is not a major complication of pure semistarvation and that the bleeding diatheses noted in the patients suffering from hunger during World War I were probably due to specific nutrient deficiencies, such as vitamin C or K.

Thus the peripheral blood in patients from the Warsaw ghetto showed a normochromic normocytic anemia, a leukopenia with a relative lymphocytosis, and a reduced platelet count. There was no relation between the magnitude of the changes in red cells, white cells, or platelets and there was little, if any, relationship between changes in any of these blood parameters and the patients' clinical condition. No evidence of specific hematologic changes such as those seen in pernicious anemia was present. None of the patients with very low white counts showed clinical evidence of granulocytopenia or agranulocytosis. One observation which was unique in this study and which has major clinical implications was that the white count showed little response to infection. Leukopenia persisted even in the face of various types of infections.

In an attempt to explain the lack of correlation of peripheral blood changes and clinical symptoms of hunger disease, the investigators examined the blood of individuals showing weight loss as their only symptom. They found similar blood changes. They conclude that it is the loss of weight itself which induces these changes. Even today we do not understand the mechanism by which semistarvation induces the changes noted in peripheral blood. Certainly even profound weight loss in obese individuals does not result in these changes. However, we still cannot exclude the possibility that weight loss in normal individuals in some way triggers the observed hematological response.

The studies performed on bone marrow were the most complete ever undertaken in living patients with hunger disease. Nine cases were studied in detail. In most, the marrow was rich in cellular elements. However, in two cases the marrow was very poor in cells. In one of these cases three attempts were unsuccessful in obtaining any marrow. In the cases containing abundant numbers of cells there was no shift toward young forms except in one case which showed a prevalence of myelocytes. No megaloblasts were observed in any of the marrows examined. In the marrows that were poor in cells a prevalence of lymphocytes was noted.

Most of the marrows showed a shift from the white cell series toward the red cell series. The authors observe that in most cases the abnormality in the marrow was a failure in normal release into the periphery rather than an abnormality in production.

A comparison of the data from the Warsaw study with that from a subsequent study on nine cases of starvation in France reported in 1948 by Lamay and co-workers reveals very similar findings. Again the shift toward red cell production is emphasized. In the Minnesota experiment only a few bone marrows were studied. The investigators observed areas of increased erythropoiesis and concluded that active red cell production was taking place.

The combined data on bone marrow changes in hunger disease would suggest that white cell production is curtailed whereas red cell production is either normal or hyperactive. This interpretation is reinforced by the observation of increased numbers of reticulocytes in some of the marrows. However, release of red blood cells into the peripheral circulation was assumed to be inhibited in some way. This inhibited release was seen as the major cause of the anemia. Another possible interpretation would involve increased destruction of red cells. This is supported by some of the findings at autopsy described in the final chapter. A number of the patients showed hemosiderin deposition in various organs. Autopsies of other patients who have died from prolonged starvation have reported similar findings. The Warsaw investigators considered this possibility but since they could not demonstrate evidence of intravascular hemolysis or of any increased tendency for red cells to hemolyze *in vitro* they discard increased destruction of red cells as a major contributor to the anemia. To me the evidence from this study and others taken together suggests that there is a combined effect of increased destruction, due primarily to a sequestration of red cells in the peripheral organs and tissues and, to a lesser extent, some difficulty in the release of red cells by the marrow. It would be extremely interesting, in view of our modern knowledge, to know the levels of erythropoietin in these patients. It is also tempting to speculate that the nature and duration of hunger and starvation are important in the ability of the marrow to respond. However, even today the reason that some patients have hypoplastic and even aplastic marrows is unexplained.

This chapter considers one aspect that could not be examined in the other studies, the effects of specific therapy. The hematology group, faced with a persistent anemia that in some cases was quite severe, administered a number of forms of therapy in an attempt to relieve this anemia. They used animal blood administered in salad, intravenous iron therapy, oral liver therapy, combined iron and liver therapy, extracts of yeast containing vitamin B, and small whole blood transfusions.

The "blood salad" had no effect; in the patients on whom it was tried the anemia continued to progress. In addition, tests on the stool demonstrated a positive benzidine reaction, the magnitude of which suggested to the investigators that a defect in intestinal absorption was present.

Oral iron was not used because it exacerbated the diarrhea; therefore, intravenous infusions of iron were tried. The side effects were numerous, and hence only two patients had the full course of six injections. No matter how the iron was administered the effect was transient. Hemoglobin rose briefly, often without any change in the red blood count. As soon as the iron therapy was discontinued the hemoglobin dropped to previous levels.

There was no response to liver therapy. The investigators point out that in spite of some similarities in the peripheral smear to pernicious anemia, the findings in the marrow, the absence of signs of hemolysis, and lack of response to specific liver therapy ruled out that diagnosis. In addition, they point out that during World War I the reports of pernicious anemia were necessarily made without bone marrow examinations or liver therapy. The peripheral findings were consistent with those in this study. They conclude that these were actually cases of the anemia of hunger disease. I should point out that at the time these observations were being made, the use of liver in the therapy for pernicious anemia was quite new and being employed in only the more advanced clinics in this country and abroad. The Warsaw investigators not only knew of this method of therapy but already had experience with it. They even knew that in some cases better results were obtained when iron and liver therapy were combined. They tried this combination in several cases with only limited success in one patient.

Although they had ruled out vitamin B complex deficiency on clinical grounds, these investigators decided on a course of B complex in the form of yeast. The results were negative in the two cases in which it was tried.

Small transfusions (120 to 200 cc) of whole blood were tried in three cases. In one the symptoms of hunger disease and the anemia were aggravated and the patient died. In the second, there was transient improvement, while in the third case the improvement was stable but other types of therapy were being employed simultaneously.

In order to verify their hypothesis that the cause of the anemia is a general food deficiency mostly due to the markedly reduced caloric intake, the investigators fed a diet with balanced nutrition and adequate calories and demonstrated improvement in all of the hematologic parameters. Unfortunately the manuscript does not give any specific details of this type of therapy. We do not know the length of refeeding or the rate of change in the hematological findings. In the Minnesota experiment this change was carefully measured. In 12 weeks of rehabilitation the increase in hemoglobin concentration observed could be entirely explained by the decrease in plasma volume which accompanied the rehabilitation. Neither supplemental vitamins nor extra protein had any effect on the rate of recovery in hemoglobin concentration. By contrast, the increase in leukocytes after 12 weeks of rehabilitation exceeded what could be accounted for by the decrease in plasma volume. This suggests a reversal in the depressed production of leukocytes described during the period of semistarvation. Hence it would appear that recovery in hemoglobin concentration is a gradual process which occurs in two phases. Initially the concentration increases as a consequence of the progressive decrease in plasma volume. This phase lasts at least 12 weeks and is unaffected by the method of refeeding. Presumably a net increase in hemoglobin occurs later. Exactly when and how this occurs is unknown. By contrast an increased rate of white cell production begins much more rapidly, and by 12 weeks a considerable increase in the concentration and total number of white cells has taken place. These data suggest that the rate of white cell production is sensitive to the caloric and protein intake of the individual. There is at present a great deal of evidence which demonstrates that in growing tissues the rate of cell division is reduced by severe malnutrition. There are other data which demonstrate that in regenerating tissue such as intestinal mucosa malnutrition can reduce the rate of cell division. Thus the data reported in the Warsaw study and in the study by Keys and co-workers are consistent with our present concepts. Cell division within the white cell series in the bone marrow is curtailed as available calories are reduced. This response is reversible and a rapid increase in the rate of cell division occurs as caloric intake is returned to normal. It is extremely interesting and somewhat surprising to me that the same response is not present in the red cell series. For some reason cell division continues at a normal and in some cases at an increased rate in the face of reduced caloric intake. Perhaps the peripheral anemia is a greater stimulus to marrow erythropoietic hyperplasia than the reduced caloric intake is to reduced cell division within the red cell series. Unfortunately the data necessary to prove this hypothesis are not currently available.

The authors conclude that all elements in the peripheral blood are reduced, resulting in a normochromic macrocytic anemia with considerable anisocytosis and poikilocytosis and an increase in reticulocytes. The leukopenia is accompanied by a relative lymphocytosis. The marrow is rich in cells with a preponderance of red cell elements. The anemia is unresponsive to all modes of specific therapy available at that time including heme iron supplied orally, nonorganic iron supplied either orally or intravenously, liver, iron and liver combined, yeast, or transfusions of whole blood. The cause of the anemia could not be ascertained but hemodilution, increased intravascular hemolysis, and decreased red cell production were all ruled out. The conclusion is that the only adequate therapy for the hematologic abnormalities is to place the patient on a diet adequate in calories and protein—the one thing that these investigators were powerless to do.

SIX Ocular Disturbances in Hunger Disease

Dr. Szymon Fajgenblat

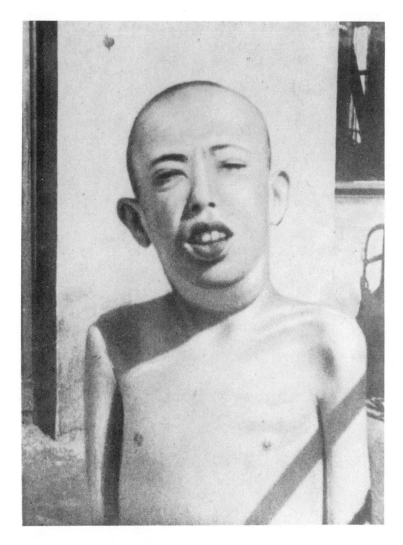

Edema of the face and neck.

W_e examined 20 young adult female patients. Unfortunately our notes and tables concerned with visual fields were lost during deportation so the exact number of certain symptoms could not be calculated.

We were not able to detect any special abnormalities or to observe any unusual complaints. We paid special attention to symptoms of night blindness, but nobody mentioned it. All through the war we saw only two patients who complained of night blindness. They were not starved but had an almost completely fat free diet. After 3 days of treatment with vitamin A their vision became normal. We will try later to explain the lack of symptoms of avitaminosis A in spite of the fat free diet of the Warsaw ghetto. We must emphasize the negative attitude of the patients toward ocular examinations and treatment. It made our work difficult and frustrating. In studying vision, especially visual fields, one has to rely on the good will and concentration of the patient.

Edema of the lids was a very common symptom. It is a sign of hunger disease, aggravated by the increased water-absorbing quality of the subdermal tissue in the eyelid. The faint lanugo covering the eyelids of some patients is also a part of the general abnormality in hair growth due to malfunction of the endocrine glands in hunger disease. Almost every patient had very long eyelashes, so characteristic of tuberculosis. We did not observe any Bitot spots or *xerosis corneae.* Conjunctivae were smooth, shiny, and clear. There were no signs of corneal malacia, which is characteristic for avitaminosis. A. Only once did we observe keratomalacia in an 18 month old baby, breast-fed by a very poorly nourished mother. Blue color of the sclera occurred in almost every patient. It could be explained by the choroid (vascular tissue) shining through thin, almost transparent sclera. The pathological complex connected with this symptom includes brittle long bones, low serum calcium, and increased excretion of calcium in the urine and feces, resulting in decalcification of the tissues. Some authors explain those symptoms by diminished efficiency of mesenchymal tissue; others consider this a secondary process bound to the decalcification. In people suffering from hunger disease the blue color of the sclera is always associated with a reduced level of calcium in blood and X-rays provide evidence of decalcification of the long bones. There were frequent fractures of the femur or collarbone, and even young people showed evidence of osteomalacia and increased bone porosity. All of these findings are signs of disturbed calcium metabolism in hunger disease. They are usually the result of dysfunction of the parathyroid glands or of vitamin D deficiency.

The pupils often contract more slowly than normal—a symptom of Adeli's syndrome. This syndrome, which is common in vitamin B deficiency, is a result of a slow neuromuscular reaction due to either low light sensitivity of the retina or weakening of the retinal muscles.

All our patients, who were young adults up to 30 years old, demonstrated early clouding of the lens similar to the changes observed in senile cataracts. Normally in this age group such clouding occurs very rarely, and then only as an inborn defect. The etiology of this type of clouding, which is very common in advancing age, is currently unknown and has been the subject of many scientific speculations. Some investigators believe it is the result of defective calcium metabolism, others, of defective water metabolism in the lens. Some investigators believe that clouding of the lens is associated with malfunction of the endocrine glands, namely hypothyroidism and hypoparathyroidism. Others believe it may be related to a lack of vitamin C. Without going into a long discussion we certainly can assume that deficient nutrition is a very important factor in early clouding of the lens.

Intraocular pressure in normal individuals measures 20 to 28 mm Hg. In certain pathological conditions the pressure is often elevated. In adrenal insufficiency or just prior to death, the pressure is very low. Our patients had low intraocular pressure, down to 12 mm Hg. Since during hunger disease blood pressure was usually low, normal levels of intraocular pressure would create too great a resistance to blood entering the retinal arteries, which would cause undernourishment of the retina and could disturb its activity. The lowering of the intraocular pressure is probably a defense mechanism preventing damage to the retina.

Almost all of our patients had normal, good eyesight, except for some incipient clouding of the lens. Examination of the fundus revealed some inadequate blood supply but no findings characteristic for a lack of vitamin A. Fields of vision examined with a light beam in daylight and nightlight and basic color discrimination (blue, red, yellow, and green) were normal.

Abnormal night vision was described a long time ago in connection with persistent hunger. Night vision is a function of rods and specifically of their light sensitive component, rodopsin, which is a derivative of vitamin A. Therefore night blindness is one of the first symptoms of vitamin A deficiency. Unfortunately we could not study night vision because of technical difficulties.

Introduction of 1:100 solution of Koch old tuberculin into the conjunctival sack in five patients resulted in a negative reaction, demonstrating anergy of the system.

Summarizing the results of our study we found the following abnormalities in people subjected to long term hunger: blue sclera, clouding of the lenses, and low intraocular pressure. These findings suggest that the real reason for the ocular and visual abnormalities in hunger disease originates in hypofunction of the thyroid, parathyroid, and adrenal glands.

We expected from our previous knowledge to find most of the changes connected with a lack of vitamin A, that is, keratomalacia, Bitot spots, *xerosis cornea,* Pillat's and night blindness. According to Pillat there is no lack of vitamin A without changes in the eye. Our findings, which differ from those of most other investigators, are even more surprising considering that our patients were deprived for years of the best sources of vitamin A, fats and egg whites.

We speculate that the absence of signs of vitamin deficiencies may be due to the fact that long lasting quantitative malnutrition somehow leads to an adjustment and a diminished requirement for vitamins. In addition, the human body tries to conserve energy in order to maintain a certain equilibrium, which may also diminish the demand for vitamins. The fact that mutual interactions occur between different vitamins suggests the possibility that similar interaction might occur between vitamins and endocrine glands.

Hypofunction of the pancreas accompanying avitaminosis B_1 and reduced blood sugar accompanying a surplus of vitamin B_1 may be examples of such interactions. It is therefore possible that hypofunction of one of the endocrine glands is acting as a defense mechanism against the lack of vitamin A.

We conclude by suggesting that the signs of vitamin deficiencies, which are characteristic in people on diets deficient in quality, do not occur in people whose diets are deficient in quantity.

EDITOR'S COMMENTS

Myron Winick, M.D.

The studies on the eye reported in this brief chapter are truly unique. They represent the most complete pathophysiologic study of ocular changes in semistarvation available on the same group of patients. This is true even though a portion of the manuscript has been lost and therefore only a summary of the visual field studies is available. To me, this chapter is very important for reasons over and above the scientific observations made by the author. Certainly, aside from the eye pathology induced by vitamin A deficiency, there was no reason to suspect that significant pathophysiologic changes in the eye would occur with semistarvation. The historical notes tell us that ocular studies were not included in the initial protocol for the investigations of hunger disease. Only later, after the studies were underway, was the author of this chapter invited to participate. Why? We can only speculate. One possibility was that some of the clinical findings in the eye were noted either by those already involved in the studies or perhaps by the ophthalmologists themselves in the course of their clinical duties. Another possibility was that the team, recognizing the availability of certain expertise and knowing that such studies had never been done, decided to take a "scientific fishing expedition" by undertaking extensive ocular investigations even though they had little hope of uncovering major pathophysiologic changes. Whatever the reason, the medical literature has been significantly enriched.

The author first addresses himself to the absence of symptoms of vitamin

A deficiency. He notes the complete absence of night blindness in the patients studied. Bitot spots, *xerosis cornea,* and corneal malacia were also absent. He concluded that even though these patients were on a very low fat intake, signs of vitamin A deficiency were not present. These observations confirmed those made by the pediatricians in children (Chapter 2). Thus vitamin A deficiency was not prevalent in any portion of the population in the Warsaw ghetto studies. The author attempts to explain the findings by postulating that prolonged caloric deprivation may reduce the requirements for vitamin A. Although we know today that this is not the only reason that vitamin A deficiency does not appear in all undernourished populations, we are still not certain whether some protection against frank signs of vitamin A deficiency may occur in calorically deprived individuals. Certain alternative explanations are possible. The most susceptible population, children under 3 years, was not studied. In fact, this population was very small because of the extremely high infant mortality and the extremely low birth rate. The population under observation had been reasonably well nourished before the war and perhaps they had stored significant amounts of vitamin A in their livers. The diet may have contained small amounts of carotene from vegetable sources, enough, however, to prevent frank deficiency symptoms from appearing. While we can only speculate at present, I suspect that all of these factors played a role in the absence of vitamin A deficiency noted in this study.

The author next turns to the positive findings uncovered in these patients. He notes edema of the eyelids and increased length of the eyelashes as part of the generalized fluid retention and hair changes in patients with hunger disease. A specific finding in the eye is blue sclerae. He explains this color as due to the choroid shining through thin, almost transparent sclera. He notes that this finding has been described in pathological conditions of bone (presumably osteogenesis imperfecta) and that in his patients it was always associated with brittle long bones, low serum calcium, increased excretion of calcium in urine and feces, and X-ray evidence of decalcification of bone. He therefore ascribes the eye finding to altered calcium metabolism. This is an interesting observation, since it has not been universally observed in patients suffering from semistarvation and may suggest some predisposing factors in the Warsaw population. The exact relationship between blue sclera and calcium metabolism, if any, is still unknown today.

The author describes sluggishly reacting pupils, which he ascribes either to a faulty retinal response to light or to sluggishly responding muscles. In view of the findings described by some of the other investigators in this study (Chapter 1) and of subsequent observations of generally poor muscle reactivity, I would tend to support the latter explanation.

A new finding at that time was the clouding of the lens in young people. The characteristics of this clouding and its progression were identical to those of senile cataracts. A number of possible causes are discussed. Today we still do not know the cause of these cataracts. It would be interesting to know whether these changes were permanent in survivors or whether nutritional rehabilitation results in reversal. It would also be extremely interesting to follow up survivors of the ghetto experience to determine if there is an increased incidence or a premature occurrence of senile cataracts in this population.

This investigator actually measured intraocular pressure in his patients. These were the first such measurements made in patients with semistarvation and to my knowledge there have been no subsequent studies of this nature. He found a marked reduction (about 50%) in intraocular pressure. He explains this as a defense mechanism to protect the retinal vessels from back pressure due to the reduced intravascular pressure. He makes no comment about the mechanism by which this reduced intraocular pressure occurs, but presumably it has something to do with the reduced arterial and venous pressures in hunger disease.

Finally, the lack of a tuberculin response, this time after insertion of old tuberculin into the conjunctival sac, is again noted.

These remarkable studies describe at least three observations which were new at that time: blue sclerae, clouding of the lens, and decreased intraocular pressure. The last, as far as I know, has not been described anywhere else in the medical literature and still awaits confirmation in other types of semistarved populations.

SEVEN Pathological Anatomy of Hunger Disease

Dr. Joseph Stein

with the collaboration of
Dr. Henryk Fenigstein

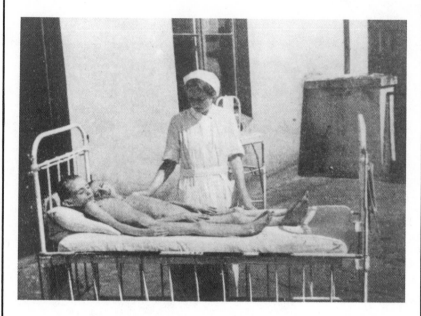

Dry cachexia in the premortal state.

S ystematic research on hunger is possible only when hunger is endemic in a large population. Massive hunger can be observed during periods of exceptional social and political upheaval, such as war or revolution. Therefore most of the major systematic studies of hunger, or rather hunger disease, originated during World War I. These studies have supplied much more extensive data than the occasional case report from which generalizations cannot be drawn and extraneous factors cannot be excluded.

Studies from World War I included for the first time a systematic description of the symptoms of different types of hunger, and contained clinical, biological, and anatomical findings. These studies allowed a number of new observations to be made, including the differentiation of a separate group of diseases caused by insufficient nutrition.

It is obvious that this group of diseases is extremely varied, depending on the quantity and quality of the diets consumed, the composition of these diets, the prevalence of hunger, and other factors. Therefore there are divergent opinions by different researchers in many areas (for example, the disagreement over the damage to blood vessels in hunger disease). Many problems still remain unsolved and their clarification requires a large amount of study.

Much of the human material from the war years 1939 to 1942 in the Warsaw ghetto is very suitable for this research, because hunger was the most significant fact of life and death (with the exception of typhus). The previous material from World War I had been collected for the most part in prisoner of war camps, since these supplied defined numbers of hungry people. In the Warsaw ghetto and especially in the centers for displaced persons, hunger reached proportions that were never before seen or heard of.

Unfortunately, the poor nutrition and poor general living conditions in the ghetto created a very difficult climate for scientific work. The lack of libraries, the lack of instruments and reagents, and the low morale associated with the constant fear of losing one's life were ever present for all. Autopsies were abundant. They should have been accompanied by histological studies. Unfortunately the work on the histopathology of hunger started only a few months before July 22, 1942, when the massive deportations started and the hospital, its institutes, laboratories, autopsy rooms, and library were completely destroyed, making any further work impossible. Up to the day of deportation, only six cases of hunger disease were examined histologically and even these were not completed—some specific studies were missing. Organs preserved in formalin were completely destroyed. Therefore the following studies do not contain the exhaustive anatomical and histological description of hunger disease that was anticipated. Instead we will present a statistical and macroscopic analysis of autopsy material.

HUNGER DISEASE AS A SEPARATE DISEASE UNIT

Diseases due to undernutrition can be divided into two groups, quantitative or caloric undernutrition and qualitative undernutrition. Often these two forms are combined, complicating the analysis of the hunger processes.

Vitamin deficiencies are a qualitative form of undernutrition and we are leaving them aside, concentrating our studies on the effects of a general lack of food.

The primary factor in hunger is the lack of nutrients that can be converted to energy. In order to obtain energy the organism uses its own organs and tissues, which eventually leads to serious disturbances. The greater the lack of food and the longer the duration of hunger, the more serious are those disturbances. Lubarsch, the author of the first known detailed anatomopathological study of hunger, divides the changes into the following groups: (1) edema, (2) scurvy, and (3) osteomalacia.

These are very different groups, both anatomically and etiologically (quantitative versus qualitative hunger). Edema as a result of long lasting caloric deficiency is the most interesting group for our study. In 1902 Wheeler described edema in prisoners of war on the island of Saint Helena. Edema was also described by many authors during and after World War I under different names, such as war dropsy, hunger dropsy, or dropsy disease. But even then some authors insisted that dropsy or edema was not always a symptom of hunger. For instance Lubarsch writes "the disease is characterised more by undernutrition than by edema," and Jackson writes in his paper on Italian war prisoners "often there are no edema signs at all." Maase-Zondeck wrote about abortive forms of hunger disease, and others "about hunger disease without edema." The most significant characteristic feature of long lasting hunger is a certain degree of cachexia, with disappearance of body fat, loss of body protein, and atrophy of many organs. These alterations are so typical and specific that unless there are other obvious reasons for cachexia they can be considered as pathognomonic for the syndrome of persistent hunger. Since the classical symptoms are also characteristic, we decided that the syndromes of changes which accompany persistent caloric deficiency should be considered a separate syndrome clinically and anatomically, which should be called hunger disease.

ANATOMICAL CHANGES IN HUNGER DISEASE

Lubarsch separates the anatomical changes in hunger disease into four groups:

1. There is a considerable disappearance of fats and lipids from the subcutaneous tissue. The fatfold thickness on the belly measures 1 to 2 mm. Sometimes it disappears completely around the internal organs, in the bone marrow, and in the adrenal cortex. (Jaffe and Sternberg described an increased amount of lipids in the adrenal cortex in their patients.) There is an increased amount of the products of fat dissocia-

tion in the lymphatic spaces around vessels in the brain and fatty droplets in the endothelium of the capillaries and in the cells of the reticuloendothelial system (RES). The adipose tissue and bone marrow have a specific jellylike appearance.

2. There is simple or brown atrophy, mostly of the heart and the liver. These organs are often very small. Heart weight is as low as 145 g and liver as low as 700 g. Even in very young people there is a large amount of lipofuscin.

3. Destruction of red blood cells and hemosiderin deposition occur in different organs. The author found them in all 55 cases examined. The localization of hemosiderin varied from individual to individual and from organ to organ. Also, the amounts deposited in various organs were different. It was most profuse in spleen, liver, kidneys, adrenals, pancreas, bone marrow, and in and around intestinal villi. It was present in epithelial and mesenchymal cells, in the reticuloendothelial system, and in striated muscle. Some authors believe the hemosiderin storage is due to blood destruction within the blood vessels and destruction of macrophages which absorb and then store this pigment. Larger localized hemosiderin deposits are due to local bleeding from capillary ruptures.

4. There is a tendency to bleeding and edema, often in the digestive tract, as described by Prym. When those changes appear in other organs, such as the lung, they lead to secondary infections, such as pneumonia.

Lubarsch considers severe damage of capillary vessels, leading to edema and petechiae, to be a very important basic symptom of hunger disease. A morphological expression of capillary damage is deposition of fat (mostly in Browicz-Kupfer liver cells and in the endothelium of intestinal capillaries). Capillary damage is also suggested by the high incidence of secondary inflammations and infections, such as lobar pneumonia and dysentery. Autopsies of patients with pneumonia often revealed bloody effusions in the lungs, purulent fibromatous inflammations of pericardium, and in 41%, concomitant purulent pneumococcal meningitis. Also in dysentery there is a tendency to effusion into serous membranes. All these symptoms strongly suggest increased permeability of capillary vessel walls.

Some authors describe considerable bleeding, which is different from scorbutic bleeding because of its small quantity and localization. Prym mentions bleeding and hemosiderin deposits in the intestinal mucosa. He believes that hemosiderosis of villi and lymph nodes is the result of blood's being absorbed from the digestive tract, and that hemosiderosis around villi and submucosa is the result of intestinal hemorrhage.

In children who died of hunger Stefko found obvious symptoms of blood diathesis. This author, looking for anatomical counterparts of the bleeding diathesis in his patients, found pathological changes in the capillary walls of the intestines and occasionally other organs. Changes consisted of swollen capillary walls, edema, and poor staining of the endothelium, often with fragmenting nuclei desquamating into the vessel lumen. There was irregular disposition of elastic fibers into the enlarged tissues of the central membrane. The lumen of vessels was much wider than expected. Stefko believes that these changes affect elasticity and contractability of vessel walls and are due to alterations in osmotic processes. This author has some very interesting conclusions in connection with the blood of people who died from hunger disease. He divides his findings into two groups:

1. Dense (thick) blood (high specific gravity, increased dry ash content, increased number of RBCs and decreased volume of plasma, changes in blood morphology), no edema, a characteristic dryness of the organs, and advanced "dry" cachexia.
2. Thin blood (low specific gravity, low amount of ash, low RBC count), edema, and dropsy.

Most of Stefko's cases belong to the first category and he believes that the first category is simply prolongation of the second, thin blood, groups. Other authors differ with this opinion. Aron states that all the organs of a hungry organism, though atrophied, are also full of water. He detects edematous changes in the later stages of hunger. Caloric hunger leads to a pathological depletion of essential substances from tissues, and by reducing plasma protein, leads to "edema-readiness." A larger water and salt intake results in frank edema in such people. Even in infants Aron describes this tendency to accumulate water, which is more marked in younger infants. Long lasting hunger in humans as well as in experimental animals results in diminished lean body mass with concomitant increased amounts of water in the organs and in the blood. In a sense, part of the tissues and organs is being replaced by water, and the loss of weight is really much greater than it appears because of the weight of the accumulated water. Our own studies have demonstrated that 1 g of lean tissue from a normal dog can be converted to 1.42 calories, whereas 1 g of tissue from a littermate on a hunger diet for 200 days is converted to only 0.55 calories. The mechanism by which edema originates in hunger disease is still unknown. Some researchers ascribe the edema to changes in the capillaries, some to diluted blood or waterlogged tissues. This probably is a very complex problem, perhaps involving certain constitutional factors in infants as well as in adults. The type of food and the increased intake of water and salt may also play a role in the formation of edema.

Druckrey studied the metabolism of isolated slices of parotid gland. He demonstrated that damaged tissue contains acid products of disintegration, which increase the osmotic pressure and enhance water retention. It is therefore possible that the acidity prevalent in hunger disease may be one of the factors involved in edema formation. Both increased and decreased water retention have been described in cold weather or after physical effort.

Since as we have stated above the etiology of hunger edema and of edema in general is not yet completely understood, many forms of idiopathic edema or edema complicating other diseases probably originate by similar mechanisms.

Experimentally one can duplicate the symptoms of hunger disease in rats by feeding them a protein deficient diet. They lose up to 46% of their body weight, display weakness, anemia, and hair loss, and in almost 50% of the animals edema occurs. In rats fed turnip peelings and margarine there is considerable fat depletion and hemosiderin is deposited in various organs.

The children are the first to show the symptoms of hunger disease, which is not surprising since children require relatively more calories than adults.

Many researchers have emphasized intestinal changes in hunger disease similar to those which occur in dysentery (excluding, of course, cases of dysentery proven bacteriologically and anatomically). The intestinal changes in dysentery are in the large intestine. They are more pronounced toward the rectum, but sometimes involve the upper part of the large intestine. These changes in hunger disease include congestion and edema of the mucous membrane, with bloody effusions and sometimes fibrous or membranous changes with necrosis. Small, superficial abscesses and, rarely, large and deep abscesses are located mostly in the lower part of the large intestine. Serological and bacteriological tests for dysentery are negative. Clinically diarrhea is present, with very profuse and frequent mucus and blood. Some researchers believe that the atrophy and edema of hunger disease are secondary to the intestinal changes. Some authors consider the intestinal changes to be derived from hunger disease because they are fresh looking and do not appear extensive enough to produce such a serious degree of cachexia. The changes described above in pseudodysentery are identical to those at the final stages of many cachexic diseases. They begin with the tendency of the edematous intestinal mucosa to become secondarily infected, possibly with normally present intestinal bacteria like E. coli. This may be due to the low resistance of cachexic patients.

In one case we were able to observe serial changes in the intestines. An original episode of bleeding caused limited necrosis with effusions until a crust was formed. When the crust was removed an abscess formed. Lately it is believed that a lack of vitamin B_2 may play a role in the pseudodysenteric changes seen in hunger disease.

Hunger osteopathy is one of the results of long term under-nutrition. It was common after the war, in 1914 through 1918, regardless of age and sex. The symptoms were present in various bones, but predominantly in the ribs, the pelvis, and the spine. There is very little anatomical information on the subject. Some authors believe the changes are characteristic for osteoporosis; others would classify the changes as osteomalacia. Some observers believe that these changes result from damage to the endocrine glands, such as enlarged parathyroids. It has been suggested that hunger osteopathy can lead to spasmophilia.

Many authors compared hunger osteopathy with the symptoms in people being fed artificially for a long time. They found hyperplastic inflammation of the bone marrow and fibrous marrow, decalcification of bones with Howship sinuses and osteoclasts, and a lack of new bone layers. These symptoms were also described in scurvy. The osteopathies are probably due not only to atrophy but also to mineral deficiency. Some researchers believe that in hunger osteopathy the changes vascillate between osteoporosis and osteomalacia. They resemble so-called porotic osteomalacia sometimes accompanied by enlarged parathyroids seen in dogs with gall bladder fistulae. However humans with similar fistulae show only porous changes in bones or may not show any skeletal changes (Mayo, Robson).

It should be clear from the above description that the symptoms of hunger disease have still not been elucidated in a completely satisfactory manner. Much additional work is indicated.

OUR MATERIAL

Our material includes 492 autopsies from January 1, 1940 until deportation on July 22, 1942, a period of about 2½ years. We tried to exclude autopsies in people who died from clearly diagnosed diseases other than hunger. The pathological anatomy department in the Jewish Hospital Czyste in Warsaw performed 3658 autopsies, of which 376 were examinations of the intestines only. Therefore the total number of complete autopsies was

TABLE 1   AUTOPSIES IN HUNGER DISEASE

Period	Total	Intestinal Autopsies	Complete Autopsies	Hunger Autopsies	Autopsies from Hunger (%)
A. January 1, 1940– December 31, 1940	768	—	768	10	1.3
B. January 1, 1941– June 30, 1941	610	5	605	101	16.7
C. July 1, 1941– December 31, 1941	1324	143	1181	246	20.8
D. January 1, 1942– July 22, 1942	956	228	728	135	18.5
Total	3658	376	3282	492	15.0

3282. Thus in 15% of our autopsies the cause of death was hunger disease.

Our material is divided into four periods: (A) January to December 1940; (B) January 1, 1941 to June 30, 1941; (C) July 1, 1941 to December 31, 1941; (D) January 1, 1942 to July 22, 1942 (Table 1).

In the later periods there are more cases of hunger disease. The increase in the number of autopsies does not depend on the number of deaths from hunger, which reached 20 to 30 daily,

TABLE 2   AGE AND SEX OF AUTOPSY MATERIAL

Age (years)	Male	Female	Total
0– 9	10	2	12
10–19	36	26	62
20–29	34	31	65
30–39	43	44	87
40–49	44	65	109
50–59	47	36	83
60–69	26	23	49
70–79	3	8	11
80–89	1	2	3
Unknown	7	4	11
Total	251 (51%)	241 (49%)	492

TABLE 3   LEVEL OF NUTRITION IN
AUTOPSIES (491 CASES)

| Nutrition | Number of Cases | | | | | Percent of Total |
	Period A	Period B	Period C	Period D	Total	
Poor	—	3	15	16	34	6.9
Very poor	4	53	83	33	173	35.2
Terrible	6	44	148	86	284	57.9

since autopsies could be performed only on the more interesting cases or those presenting diagnostic problems.

Table 2 shows that our material is composed of mainly middle aged people of both sexes. Table 3 demonstrates the severity of malnutrition in our cases. Table 4 differentiates patients on the basis of color changes in the skin. There were two types of patient: those whose color was pale, almost cadaverlike, and those whose skin color was dark brown. The latter group comprised only 17.5%.

Table 5 contains data on edema and effusions into serous cavities. Edema was present in about one third of the cases. It was most frequent in the lower extremities. The trunk and upper extremities were rarely affected. Effusions were most frequently observed in the abdominal cavity.

From Table 6 it is clear that edema appears most often in people with pale skin; only 13.8% of the cases had dark or brown skin. However, pale skin also occurs in cases of "dry atrophy" (Table 7). By contrast, since from a total of 81 cases with brown skin (Table 4) only 20 had edema and 61 had "dry

TABLE 4   SKIN COLOR IN DEATH FROM HUNGER
DISEASE (466 CASES)

| Color | Number of Cases | | | | | Percent of Total |
	Period A	Period B	Period C	Period D	Total	
Pale, cadaverlike	5	85	202	93	385	82.5
Dark, brown	—	13	28	40	81	17.5

TABLE 5 FREQUENCY AND LOCALIZATION
OF EDEMA IN HUNGER DISEASE

	Number of Cases				
	Period	Period	Period	Period	
Localization	A	B	C	D	Total
Torso	—	1	10	7	18
Upper extremities	—	1	14	6	21
Lower extremities	3	18	95	41	157
Autopsies with	3	34	91	32	160
Generalized edema	30	33.6	38.6	30.4	32.5
edema (%)					

TABLE 6 HUNGER EDEMA AND SKIN
COLOR (145 CASES)

	Number of Cases					
	Period	Period	Period	Period		Percent
Color	A	B	C	D	Total	of Total
Pale	1	17	83	24	125	86.2
Brown	—	1	7	12	20	13.8

TABLE 7 "DRY" ATROPHY AND SKIN
COLOR (321 CASES)

	Period					Percent
Color	A	B	C	D	Total	of Total
Pale	4	68	119	69	260	81.0
Brown	—	12	21	28	61	19.0

atrophy" (Table 6), one must conclude that dark skin rarely accompanies edema and is prevalent in "dry atrophy."

In Table 8 we present the frequency of atrophy of various organs. In agreement with other researchers we observed that heart, liver, spleen, and kidney undergo atrophy regularly. The latest period in 1942 shows heart atrophy in 89%, liver atrophy in 87.5%, and spleen and kidney atrophy in 82.4% of hunger disease autopsies.

Table 9 shows that the weight of the brain is unchanged,

TABLE 8   ATROPHY OF ORGANS IN HUNGER DISEASE

Organ	Number of Cases of Atrophy				
	Period A	Period B	Period C	Period D	Total
Heart					
Total	6 (60%)	83 (82.2%)	210 (85.4%)	120 (89%)	419 (85%)
Brown	5	47	78	76	206
Liver					
Total	6 (60%)	81 (80.2%)	209 (85.3%)	118 (87.5%)	414 (84%)
Brown	2	54	91	76	223
Kidneys	6 (60%)	77 (76.2%)	196 (79.7%)	111 (82.4%)	390 (79.3%)
Spleen	6 (60%)	77 (76.2%)	198 (80.5%)	111 (82.4%)	392 (79.7%)

whereas heart, liver, kidney, and spleen are considerably lighter (sometimes as low as 40 g for spleen and 65 g for kidneys). We compare our specimens to normal values developed by Professor L. Paszkiewicz and reported in his book *Technique of Autopsies.*

Table 10 demonstrates the degree of atrophy of skeletal muscles. Only 2.7% could be classified normal. In Table 11 we summarize the intestinal changes in autopsied cases of hunger disease. These changes were present in 27.2% of all cases. The most important findings were edema and reddish discoloration of the mucosa, with a variable amount of mucus present. Some

TABLE 9   WEIGHT OF ORGANS IN HUNGER DISEASE (FROM AUTOPSIES OF PERSONS 20–60 YEARS OLD)

Organ	Weight Recorded in Autopsies (g)			Normal Weight[a] (g)
	Average	Smallest	Biggest	
Brain	1309	760	1680	1310
Heart	220	110	350	275
Liver	865	545	1600	1500–2000
Kidney				
Right	112	70	190	150
Left	114	65	190	155
Spleen	103	40	310	150–250

[a] As reported in L. Paszkiewicz, *Technique of Autopsies.*

TABLE 10   DEVELOPMENT OF SKELETAL MUSCLES
(359 CASES)

| Level of Development | Number of Cases | | | | | Percent of Total |
	Period A	Period B	Period C	Period D	Total	
Poor	8	44	103	64	219	61.0
Fair	2	42	37	49	130	36.3
Good	—	—	5	5	10	2.7

of these changes are part of the picture of edema as seen in the edema of subcutaneous tissue or in the skin itself.

Table 12 confirms findings of other researchers that in 77.7% of people who died from hunger, bile is watery and thin.

Table 13 confirms findings of other researchers that in 50% of the cases there is considerable reduction in the number of fat bodies in the adrenals.

Table 14 unfortunately summarizes only nine cases; however seven of them showed a jellylike consistency of the bone marrow.

Table 15 summarizes the results of the study on the cases of emphysema that occurred in hunger disease. In 370 cases where detailed lung study was conducted there were 13.8% with emphysema. Although the changes were present mostly in young adults they resembled those of emphysema of old age. Since these changes probably represent atrophy of the lungs, analogous to atrophic changes in other organs, hunger emphysema should be considered "involuted" edema.

TABLE 11   CHANGES
IN THE INTESTINES

Period	Number of Cases
A	5
B	21
C	66
D	41
Total	133 (27.2%)

TABLE 12 DENSITY OF BILE IN HUNGER
DISEASE (121 CASES)

| | Number of Cases | | | | | |
Density	Period A	Period B	Period C	Period D	Total	Percent of Total
Thin	2	27	20	45	94	77.7
Thick	2	6	6	13	27	22.3

TABLE 13 AMOUNT OF FAT IN ADRENALS IN
HUNGER DISEASE (285 CASES)

Period	Number of Adrenals	Number with Low Lipids	Cases with Low Lipids (%)
A	10	7	70
B	89	55	61.9
C	71	20	28.2
D	115	58	50.5
Total	285	140	49.2

TABLE 14 BONE MARROW IN
DEATH FROM HUNGER DISEASE
(9 CASES)

Color and Texture	Number of Cases
Yellow	2
Yellow, jellylike	3
Pink, jellylike	1
Red, jellylike	1
Raspberry, jellylike	2

Petechiae occur very rarely. They are present mostly in the intestinal mucosa. In one case we observed larger petechiae in the skin and in another case in the adrenals (connected with clots in the adrenal veins; see summary of histological findings below). General anemia was found in only 27 cases, or 5.5%.

We would like to draw special attention to the intestinal changes, which simulated dysentery. They are presented in Table 16. At the beginning of our study we believed this to be real dysentery, but bacteriological and serological studies of the

TABLE 15   FREQUENCY OF
EMPHYSEMA IN HUNGER
DISEASE (370 CASES)

Age (years)	Number of Cases
0– 9	1
10–19	3
20–29	10
30–39	6
40–49	14
50–59	8
60–69	6
70–79	1
80–89	1
Total	50 (13.5%)

intestinal content were negative for dysentery. Gradually we observed symptoms that were less characteristic for dysentery (for example, small branlike fibrous infiltrations in the mucosa and small superficial ulcerations). These changes were obviously freshly acquired, probably in the last days or weeks of life. In real dysentery the changes were extensive, resulting from the long duration of the disease. Therefore, we decided that the symptoms in patients with hunger disease were rather pseudodysentery, as described by many authors during World War I.

Since we had 218 cases of severe intestinal disturbances, we decided to devote a separate chapter to this subject. Unfortunately it was not finished in time to be included here.

TABLE 16   DATA ON CACHEXIA WITH
PSEUDODYSENTERY, ATROPHY, AND EDEMA

Period	Pseudodysentery (Total)		Atrophy		Edema	
	Number of Cases	%	Number of Cases	%	Number of Cases	%
A	16	2.1	12	75.0	4	25.0
B	48	8.0	29	60.0	21	44.0
C	113	9.5	79	70.0	55	48.5
D	41	5.6	19	46.0	20	49.0
Totals	218	5.9	139	63.7	100	45.8

We will add here that the cases described as pseudodysentery are cases of hunger disease complicated by intestinal symptoms that etiologically have no connection with dysentery. Therefore we have called them pseudodysentery. They probably result from secondary infection of the edematous and bloated intestinal mucosa or from toxic products secondary to metabolic disturbances which act on the intestinal mucosa in a manner similar to uremia.

In 63.7% of the cases of hunger disease with pseudodysenteric changes in the intestine, we found atrophy of various organs, and 45.8% of the cases were edematous.

HISTOLOGY

In only six cases are histological studies available and these were not investigated as completely as they should have been. Four cases are strictly hunger disease and two cases are complicated by pseudodysentery. A summary of these is included below.

Summary of Histological Findings

Three males and three females 16 to 42 years old were studied. In one of them symptoms suggesting typhus were found in the brain, but we included this one in this summary because of its typical atrophy of hunger disease. We also had very limited material to present. In histological evaluation the atrophy is predominant, as shown in Table 17. Large quantities of hemosiderin were present in liver and spleen. In lungs it was rare or present only in very small amounts.

The following is a summary of findings in the endocrine glands.

1. Pancreas. Numerous islands of Langerhans with insignificant symptoms of atrophy (nuclear pycnosis). In two of the five cases examined, small vacuole changes. In three cases islands looked like tubes.

2. Adrenals. In two cases there were fat bodies. In one case parietal thrombosis in veins, petechiae, necrosis. In three cases no pathological changes.
3. Thyroid. Normal in four cases.
4. Parathyroid. Normal in five cases.
5. Pituitary. Generally normal. In four cases out of five examined the central part was poorly developed. In two cases posterior part had many cells with brown pigment and free strewn pigment. In two cases prevalence of eosinophils over basophils. In one case very few basophil cells.
6. Testes. Atrophy in two cases out of three examined. Very few Leydig's cells in all three cases.
7. Ovaries. Atrophy in one case out of three examined.
8. Epiphysis. Normal with few calcifications in all four cases.

TABLE 17   SUMMARY OF HISTOLOGICAL FINDINGS

Number of Cases	Organ	Findings
6	Cardiac muscle	4 cases brown atrophy
5	Lungs	All cases emphysematic changes
6	Spleen	All cases atrophy, 4 cases examined for hemosiderin, 1 small amount, 3 cases large amounts
6	Skin	5 cases much melanin and many chromatophores, little keratohyalin. In 4 cases small clusters of lymphocytes around blood vessels in dermis. Slight papillar layer
6	Kidneys	5 cases hyaline drops in epithelium of curved canals. In 2 cases effusion liquid in Bowman's capsulae
4	Liver	4 cases typical brown atrophy. In 2 cases examined for hemosiderin much was found. In 1 case mostly within the liver cells
5	Pancreas	1 case of atrophy
3	Testes	2 cases of atrophy
3	Ovaries	1 case of atrophy
2	Lymphatic glands	1 case of atrophy
4	Striped muscle	2 cases of atrophy
3	Bone marrow	3 cases of atrophy
2	Nipple	2 cases of atrophy

DISCUSSION

Our material contained 492 cases of hunger disease without complications—15% of all complete autopsies—and 218 cases of hunger disease with pseudodysentery in intestines—5.9% of all completed autopsies.

According to our findings, which are in agreement with those of other authors, the most important changes in hunger disease are complete atrophy of adipose tissue and atrophy of organs with concomitant advanced cachexia. Of our cases, 57.9% were very poorly nourished. Heart, liver, kidneys, and spleen were most atrophic. Their weight was very low; the lowest for heart was 110 g, for liver 545 g, for kidney 65 to 70 g, for spleen 40 g, and for brain 760 g. Skeletal muscles were also largely atrophic. The number of fatty bodies in adrenals was very low under macroscopic examination in half our cases. Bone marrow, regardless of its color, looked like jelly.

Considering that a hungry organism, no matter how economically functioning, does not receive enough calories from outside, these atrophic changes are understandable. The body uses first the accumulated and stored fat, and then burns its own tissues. Therefore atrophy appears. We lack here measurements of glycogen in liver and in muscles.

The typical anatomical picture of death from hunger, when added to the specific clinical symptoms, allows one to differentiate hunger disease as a separate entity.

Age and sex do not influence the origin and course of hunger disease. We must emphasize that only 5.5% of the cases showed advanced anemia. Fairly large amounts of hemosiderin are found in livers and spleens, and it is certain that in hunger disease RBCs are being destroyed, but on the other hand as a result of the diminished size of organs and tissues, the amount of blood left is enough to prevent the symptoms of advanced anemia. In hunger disease autopsies, bile was thin and watery.

Edema

Of 160 cases, 32.5% showed edema and effusions, mostly edema of the lower extremities and effusions into serous cavities.

The mechanism of edema is not yet quite clear. We know that in most cases the tissues retain water, but this symptom is again dependent on many factors. Tissue acidosis is one of them, with hydrogen ions acting by osmosis to increase absorption of water by the tissue colloids, which results in water retention and edema. It is also possible that an increase in ingested water and salt and certain constitutional factors are involved in the pathogenesis of the edema.

The observation that physical effort and cold increase edema is easy to explain. Physical effort acidifies the tissues, making them retain more water. Cold temperature increases the permeability of capillary walls. This last possibility can play a role in the formation of edema. Some authors believe that this permeability is the most important factor in the process of forming edema.

It is interesting that people with brownish skin are usually subject to "dry" cachexia without edema. Maybe this is connected with some constitutional factors promoting water absorption and preventing its loss through tissues.

Color of Skin

In spite of the fact that histological examination detected melanin in many cases, we found that dark skin was present only in 19% of the cases, and pale skin in 81%. But there is a relationship between brownish dark skin and "dry" cachexia. In 81 cases of brown skin, 61 had dry cachexia and only 20 had edema.

Emphysema

Emphysema was found in 50 cases out of 370 examined, or 13.5%. The emphysematous changes were spontaneous or looked like old age emphysema in spite of the general youth of patients. Emphysema in hunger disease is probably due to atrophic changes in the lungs analogous to changes in other organs. Therefore it should be considered as involution edema.

Bleeding

We saw only two cases of bleeding besides minor intestinal bleeding or more serious bleeding due to pseudodysentery. Other authors write about bleeding in hunger disease, but they probably included cases of avitaminosis, which are excluded from our study.

Catarrhal and Edematous Changes in the Intestines

The most common change was gastritis connected with edema of the mucosa. It is possible that this is one more symptom of edema involving the whole organism.

Pseudodysentery Changes in the Intestines

We separated from our material 218 cases of hunger disease with symptoms of dysentery. They have to be considered as complications of hunger disease or as secondary infection of bloated and edematous intestinal mucosa or mucosa damaged by toxic products of defective metabolism in hunger disease. These changes in the intestines are similar to those in uremia, for example. They have no connection with dysentery and are only superficially anatomic; therefore we call them pseudodysentery.

Hunger Osteopathy

The material we collected was destroyed completely. In three autopsies we observed advanced osteoporosis. From data lost from the surgery department we know that unfortunately the breaking of bones was very widespread, especially the neck of the femur, and the surgeons commented on the poor quality of bone tissue, which made healing very difficult and pinning almost impossible. In one case we examined the remnants of such a break. It showed osteoporosis with decalcification, and therefore the changes could be classified between osteomalacia and osteoporosis. Probably hunger osteopathy is not an anatomoclinical entity. Different symptoms were described, all derived from undernutrition, from simple atrophic osteoporosis, to different types of atrophy and decalcification, up to complete osteomalacia and eventually rachitism. Hunger osteopathy is probably one more symptom of general atrophy.

Undernutrition and Amyloidosis

We were surprised at the rarity of amyloidosis in our autopsy material—only six cases. We would have expected it to appear quite often because of so much tuberculosis and chronic purulent processes. Perhaps very virulent tuberculosis progressed so fast that there was no time for the development of amyloidosis.

We believe that the absence of amyloidosis in our material is due to the lack of protein in the food, mostly proteins which are essential for amyloid formation (according to Kuczynski) for example, egg albumin and milk.

Japanese authors (see Tanaka) believe that the rarity of amyloidosis in the Japanese people is the result of insufficient protein in their diet.

EDITOR'S COMMENTS

Myron Winick, M.D.

This chapter describes in detail the post-mortem findings in patients who died of hunger disease. The author begins by reviewing the literature up to that time. He points out that even during World War I, complete pathological studies were not available because of the lack of proper equipment in the prisoner of war camps. However, it was noted at that time that two types of malnutrition occurred, the first due to qualitative abnormalities in the diet, such as vitamin deficiencies, and the second due to quantitative deficiency, or semistarvation. Since the type of deficiency seen in the Warsaw ghetto was semistarvation, he limits further discussion to that form of malnutrition. The author of this chapter and his collaborator were aware of the literature on hunger edema and of the controversy in the medical literature over whether all patients suffering from semistarvation had some degree of tissue edema. Therefore, they focused their own research on this problem. They note that some authors divided patients by whether the blood had a high or low specific gravity, those with high specific gravity having tissues which were dehydrated and hence having a dry or cachexic form of semistarvation. By contrast, in patients whose blood was of low specific gravity, the tissues were waterlogged and the patients had edema. Other authors disagreed with this point of view, stating that even in tissues which were markedly atrophic, from patients with no clinical edema, the percentage of water is increased. The authors of this chapter agree with the second point of view and discuss some experimental work of their own in which they were able to demonstrate that whereas 1 g of lean tissue from a normal dog could be converted to 1.42 calories, 1 g of lean tissue from a littermate on a prolonged restricted diet (200 days) could be converted to only 0.55 calories. They concluded that the noncaloric component of the lean tissue was additional water. In addition, they state that in rats placed on a protein restricted diet, 50% developed edema. These studies are extremely interesting and I should like to know whether they had been published. The authors had apparently produced experimental kwashiorkor in dogs and rats. Later investigators have had great difficulty in devising an animal model for this disease. Perhaps if the exact methods employed by these investigators were known, the search for this model might have ended successfully much earlier.

Prior reports had classified the anatomical changes in patients who died of semistarvation into four categories:

1. Disappearance of fat from the subcutaneous and deep depots.
2. Simple or brown atrophy, most marked in heart and liver.
3. Destruction of red blood cells, with hemosiderin deposits in tissues, particularly in spleen, liver, kidney, adrenals, pancreas, bone marrow, and intestinal villi.
4. A tendency to hemorrhage and edema of the gastrointestinal tract.

The authors of this chapter paid special attention to these characteristics in their own studies. Two other types of changes that had been previously described in hunger disease are discussed in some detail. The changes in the gastrointestinal tract include congestion and edema of the mucous membrane, blood effusions, and often fibrous or membranous changes, with occasional necrosis. They note the difficulty in differentiating these changes from those found in dysentery of infectious origin. However, they believe the distinction can be made on pathologic findings and by using culture techniques. They call the symptoms in pure hunger disease pseudodysentery.

The second change associated with prolonged semistarvation that they discuss is "hunger osteopathy." They point out that this syndrome was very common during World War I and that symptoms were present mostly in the ribs, pelvis, and spine. They also point out that there was very little anatomical information about the nature of the bone abnormalities in semistarvation. Some authors reported the lesions of osteoporosis, others osteomalacia. Some found hyperplastic inflammation of bone marrow, whereas others reported fibrous marrow. There were also reports of marked decalcification of bone.

Thus, these investigators began their studies well aware of the preceding literature and of the most important questions that still remained unanswered. They report on 492 autopsies performed in the 2½ years that preceded the deportations. These were cases of "pure" hunger disease with no other complications. This represented about 15% of the total number of autopsies performed in their department during the same period. They divided their material into four periods beginning in January 1940 and ending on July 22, 1942, and point out that the number of cases of hunger disease increased with time.

In a series of tables the authors document the following gross changes:

1. Pale cadaverlike skin in 82.5% of the cases. Dark brown colored skin in 17.5%.
2. Edema in one third of the cases. Effusions were most frequent in the abdominal cavity when they occurred.
3. Edema was rare in cases of "brown skin," whereas the pale skin group had either the edematous or the dry form of the disease.
4. Severe atrophy occurred in heart, liver, spleen, and kidney.
5. Brain weight remained unchanged (these were adult patients).
6. Marked skeletal muscle atrophy.
7. Edema of the small intestinal wall with swollen reddish discolored mucosa and mucus appeared in 27.2% of the cases.
8. Thin watery bile in 77.7% of cases.
9. Reduced number of fat bodies in the adrenals in 50% of cases.
10. Jellylike consistency in bone marrow of certain cases.
11. Emphysema in 13.8% of cases.
12. Anemia in only 5.5% of cases.
13. Almost 50% of the cases had intestinal changes that could be classified as pseudodysentery. An equal number of these cases fell into the edematous and nonedematous groups.

These data include a number of interesting observations about which we can only speculate even today. The brown skin in almost 20% of the patients, coupled with the gross findings of adrenal atrophy in many of the patients, suggest that some of the patients may have had a form of Addison's disease. This is speculated about in the chapter on clinical signs and further strengthened by the autopsy data. However, the limited number of histologic observations on the adrenals (six cases) failed to substantiate this diagnosis. Only two of these cases, however, had brown skin, and hence it is difficult to draw any conclusions. The observation that brown skin was rarely accompanied by edema is certainly intriguing, but I must confess I have no idea what this might signify. The observations on the brain sparing were not new in adults. Unfortunately, the authors do not mention whether brain weight was more affected in children if death occurred early enough. I doubt if these data were available in this study, since young infants were excluded. However, it is possible that these data were present in the general autopsy material.

The high prevalence of emphysema in young adult patients is an interesting observation and, in my opinion, was better demonstrated in this study than in any previous or subsequent study. The low incidence of severe anemia contradicted many previous reports but has been substantiated by many subsequent studies, including those of Keys and co-workers.

Unfortunately, only six cases were studied histologically, owing to the short duration of the study and the lack of equipment. The only consistent findings were the deposition of hemosiderin in liver and spleen, atrophy and decreased number of Leydig's cells in testis, and atrophic changes in other organs. These findings confirmed previous observations, but the detailed data that the authors hoped to obtain in order to answer some of the questions that they pose at the beginning of their chapter was unfortunately not forthcoming. Thus, the chapter represents a remarkable cataloguing of the gross anatomical changes in hunger disease, but the histologic alterations producing these changes unfortunately could not be documented.

APPENDIX

Autopsy Reports of Individual Cases

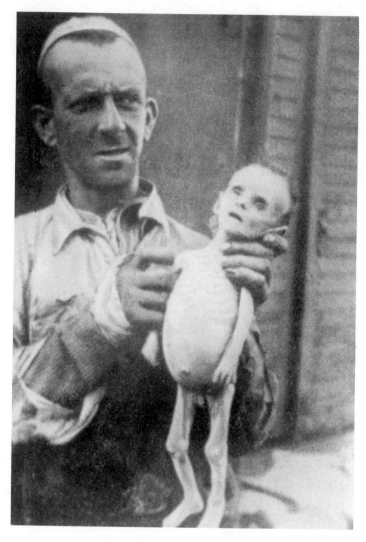

Severe marasmus and death.

CASE 1

Male, 32 years old, 49 hours after death. Clinical diagnosis: advanced inanition. Anatomopathological diagnosis: inanition and atrophy of the organs; bleeding into the right adrenal, hydropericardium, and hydrothorax; bilateral ascites; edema of the legs and feet; emphysema and edema of the lungs.

From the Autopsy Report

Height above average, very poorly nourished, build normal; hair light brown. Skin cadaverlike, pallid, rather elastic; small scars on the abdomen; edema on the legs and feet. Abdomen about 250 ml, pleural cavity about 600 ml, pericardial sack 50 ml of fluid. Heart the size of a fist, weight 220 g; no macroscopic changes, except sclerotic islands in the aorta. Lungs rather large, meeting borders, poor elasticity, full of air, grey-pink-black, partially bloated. Spleen fluffy, atrophic, weight 90 g. Adrenals normal, right 15 g, left 13.75 g. In the capsule, mostly on the right, there were several bloody effusions. The cortex was narrow and light yellow; the medulla was narrow and greyish in color. Kidneys slightly atrophic, right 160 g, left 140 g, otherwise normal. Liver brown atrophy, 1300 g. Stomach and intestines normal. Brain macroscopically normal, weight 1300 g.

Microscopic Study

Brain: normal architecture, vessels full of blood, epiphysis normal with numerous calcifications.

Stomach: many lymphocytes on the surface of the mucosa. In some places large lumps of mucus full of lymphocytes and leukocytes adhering to the mucosa.

Cardiac muscle: normal. In spots small smudges of fibrous connective tissue, and muscular fragmentation.

Spleen: capsule and trabeculae thick, glassy; vessel walls thick, glassy; lumen narrow. In the red pulp there is a growth of reticulum. Vessels and sinuses are profusely filled with blood. Lymph nodes very small, not well differentiated from their surroundings.

Skin: epidermis very thin, slight papillary layer, increased pigmentation in the epidermis. Increased number of pigment carrying cells in the dermis. Horny layer thin in some parts and thick in others. The dermis is made up of slightly bloated loose connective tissue.

Kidneys: normal. Small glomerulae with numerous nuclei. Canaliculi normal; slight mesenchymal changes in epithelium. Vessels filled with blood.

Liver: normal. Hyperemic from large vessels to small capillaries. In many places, but primarily around the central veins, there were bloody discharges.

Pancreas: shrunken ascinae and empty ducts, some with sunken walls. Numerous, usually small, islands of Langerhans made up of different sized cells, many with pyknotic darkly staining nuclei. Cytoplasm in these cells is often invisible and there are often vacuolelike spaces between cells. In some islands these empty spaces predominate.

Thyroid: formed with normal or slightly larger alveolae filled with neutral or eosinophilic colloid. Sometimes there are smudgelike aggregations of round cells with darkly staining nuclei and sparse cytoplasm between the alveolae.

Adrenals: the cortex is almost totally necrotic, partly infiltrated with blood, and, in some areas, small granular looking bodies. In the medulla around the entire gland there were several large areas of hemorrhage. Blood vessels were full of blood, some partially or completely occluded with thrombi. In some places there are leukocytes and fibroblasts extending from the capsule into necrotic tissue.

Pituitary: the frontal lobe contains a variety of cells; in some places eosinophils prevail, in some basophils, in some principals. In the median part there are a few encapsulated bodies lined mostly with principal cells and occasionally with eosinophils. The posterior lobe is normal, containing considerable amounts of melanin, and in the part which adjoins the anterior lobe there are small groups of both eosinophils and basophils.

Testes: the sperm ducts are separated from each other by bundles of compact connective tissue. The ducts contain spermatogenic cells. In some places in the connective tissue between the ducts there are small groups of two to three parenchymal cells with brown pigment.

This case shows general atrophy of organs. The major findings are thromboses, petechiae, necrotic changes in the adrenal cortex (probably the cause of death), and pulmonary emphysema.

CASE 2

Female, 16 years old, 18 hours after death. Clinical diagnosis: inanition, acute enterocolitis. Anatomopathological diagnosis: advanced inanition, atrophy of organs, brown atrophy of the liver and myocardium. Nodular tuberculosis of the left pleura. Serofibrinous pleuritis on both sides. Tuberculous lymphadenitis, ascites, edema of the feet and ankles. Enterocolitis, catarrhalis, ascaris lumbricoides in the esophagus. Third degree bed sores on the trochanter, the iliac crest, and the sacrum.

From the Autopsy Report

Height below average, very poorly nourished, fragile build. Hair light brown. Skin thin, swarthy, nonelastic, desquamations on the abdomen and chest. Brain 1300 g, very soft, bloated. Macroscopically normal in the vascular meninx. On the base of the brain there is a small amount of clear liquid. In the abdominal cavity there are about 2 liters of clear yellow liquid; in the right pleura 900 ml, and in the left 1 liter of clear yellow liquid. There is a small fibrous growth on the posterior pleural surface. On the left pleural surface there are several lentil sized whitish tumors. Heart 150 g; smaller than the fist of the deceased. Fifty ml of percolated liquid in the pericardium. Cavities usual width, valves small and smooth. Cardiac muscle normal, brown in color, and solid to palpation. The right atrium was 0.1 cm thick; the left atrium was 0.8 cm thick. The lungs were small, light, fluffy, and a pale greyish pink color. The glands in the hilus of the lungs were of normal size and contained several large whitish tumors. The spleen was atrophied, 120 g, with a small scar close to the lower border. Adrenals were flat, with no macroscopic changes. The kidneys were atrophic, weighing 100 g each. The liver showed brown atrophy and weighed 800 g. The stomach was small and empty with smooth yellowish grey-pink mucosa. The sex organs were normal. The intestinal mucosa was bloated and covered with greyish and yellowish mucus.

Microscopic Study

Brain: normal architecture. Two types of changes in the vessels: deposition of hyaline within the adventitia, and focal infiltrations with lymphocytes and large round cells with large uniformly colored nuclei and very little cytoplasm. In some small vessels there are hyaline thrombi. In the spaces between the vessels there are several areas of finely granulated brown pigment. The vascular meninx is thick and bloated, and contains scattered usually single round large cells, with dark uniformly colored nuclei and very little cytoplasm.
   Cerebellum and medulla oblongata: normal.
   Cardiac muscle: the fibers are thin and lipofuscin surrounds the nuclei. Between the fibers there are patches of loose or compact connective tissue with a large number of lymphocyte-like cells or oblong cells with band shaped nuclei.
   Aorta: normal.
   Lungs: alveolar structure is normal; however in places the alveoli are quite large with very thin walls. Some alveoli contain some seral liquid cells, lymphocytes, and cells containing coal dust. In some bronchiae there are numerous macrophages or large lymphocytes and clumps of bacteria. Larger areas of lymphocyte infiltration are present in or under the pleura. The iron test is negative.

Spleen: numerous small Malpighi nodules, with narrow lumens and hyaline changes in the vessels. The capsule and trabecule are thick. In the red pulp there is a profuse reticulum and very profuse hemosiderin deposits, mostly in the walls of the sinuses and in reticular cells. Many cells loaded with hemosiderin are in the lumen of blood vessels. Some red blood cells contain nuclei.

Skin: thin epidermis with a large amount of melanin in the basal cell layer. The lower layers of epidermis are not well separated from the connective tissue of the dermis. There is extensive cornification, which is not uniform, and certain areas contain dispersed keratohyaline. The papillary layer is thin. There are many cells containing melanin in the connective tissue under the epidermis and around vessels. There are small groups of lymphocytes of tunica adventitial origin.

Kidneys: normal.

Liver: thin trabecule. Intratrabecular spaces full of serum, with areas containing single lymphocytic cells. Small lipofuscin granules randomly dispersed in the cytoplasm of cells in the central lobule. In Kernan cavities there is extensive infiltration, mostly with lymphocytes. In the small intralobular vessels there are numerous hyaline changes. In one spot there is a nonspecific papule. Moderate diffuse hemosiderosis with iron deposited in liver cells and in fibrocytes in the central parts or around the lobule.

Adrenals: flattened, their glomerular layer with a well differentiated band shaped layer and slightly widened reticular layer. In the glomerular and band shaped layer the cells have regular foamy cytoplasm. There is little pigment in the reticular layer. Medullary layer is underdeveloped, with many groups of cortical cells.

Thyroid: large and medium sized spaces filled with acidophilic colloid. The walls of the alveolae are thin.

Parathyroids: some cells contain vacuoles and in some areas there are glandular bodies.

Pituitary: normal.

Epiphysis: contains a small amount of calcium deposits,

mostly in the capsule. In the central part there is a good sized cavity containing liquid serum.

Ovaries: large with numerous young oocytes, whitish bodies, and a few mature graffian follicles. In some areas there are small groups of roundish or oval cells with cytoplasm full of brown pigment.

Striated muscle: normal.

Bone marrow: fibrous and sparsely cellular. The cells present are mostly myeloblasts and myelocytes, with a few leukocytes and cells with round nuclei. In spots there are cells with red nuclei.

The characteristics of this case are atrophy of the organs, and large amounts of hemosiderin in the liver and even in the liver cells and in the spleen.

CASE 3

Male, 23 years old, autopsy after 50 hours. Clinical diagnosis: inanition, enterocolitis. Anatomopathological diagnosis: advanced inanition, atrophy of the organs, purulent diffuse bronchitis, botriocephalus in the small intestine.

From the Autopsy Report

Medium height, normal build, poor nutrition, black hair, elastic, thin, and swarthy skin. Lack of edema, normal brain, weight 1260 g. Small pleural effusion. Heart the size of the deceased's fist, smooth thin valves, atria of normal width. Cardiac muscle normal, pinkish brown, dense. Thickness of left atrium 0.8 cm, of right 0.1 cm. Normal sized lungs collapsing normally. When cut, full of air. Bright red bronchi containing drops of mucopurulent liquid. Small atrophic spleen; normal sized flat adrenals, very narrow cortex, yellowish color, very narrow greyish medulla. Small atrophic kidneys. Small brown atrophic liver. Sex organs, stomach, and intestines normal, except for the parasite botriocephalus in the small intestine.

Microscopic Study

Cardiac muscle: normal. Thin fibers with large hyperchromic nuclei.

Spleen: thickened capsule and partially hyalinized trabeculae. Small lymph nodes, sparsely scattered, uneven in shape, and without proliferating foci. Their vessels have thick hyaline walls with narrow lumens. In the red pulp there is increased reticulum. Pigment containing iron is present in red pulp, in reticulum cells, and in the surrounding cavities.

Skin: thin epithelium. In spots only three or four layers of cells are well differentiated. In the basal layer there is profuse melanin. The granular layer is underdeveloped. In spots there is keratohyaline and the keratin layer is medium thick. The papillary layers are hardly noticeable. The cutis mostly just below the epithelium contains many melanin carrying cells and free melanin bodies. Deeper there are small lymphocyte infiltrations, probably of tunica adventitial origin, around capillaries.

Kidneys: small glomeruli containing blood. In spots there are clusters of leukocytes with single nuclei. The curved tubules have thin walls and broad lumens. In the epithelium there were small hyaline drops. The blood supply appeared adequate.

Liver: thin trabeculae separated by wide crevices full of blood. In the liver cells there are small amounts of finely granulated brown pigment. In spots the cells contain large hyperchromic nuclei. Some cells have two nuclei. There are lymphocytes in Kernan's cavities. The iron test demonstrates many iron granules in the cytoplasm of liver cells, sometimes in fibrocytes.

Pancreas: normal architecture. Islands of Langerhans composed of cells of different sizes, from very small with dark uniform nuclei to large with alveolar or hyperchromic nuclei. Cytoplasm, not always visible, sometimes contains vacuoles.

This is a case of organ atrophy with large amounts of hemosiderin.

CASE 4

Female, 18 years old, 16 hours after death. Clinical diagnosis: inanition, acute enterocolitis, edema of the extremities. Anatomopathological diagnosis: extensive inanition, anemia, and atrophy of the organs, emphysema in upper part of the lungs, edema in the lower part. Ascites, edema of the face, edema of extremities. Fatty bone marrow from the right femur. Thyroid adenomatous, gastroenterocolitis, cholelithiasis.

From the Autopsy Report

Build normal, height below average, nutrition very poor, hair light brown. Skin dirty grey, yellowish on the chest and back, brownish face, edema of soles and outside of hands. Brain normal architecture, weight 1180 g. In the abdominal cavity there are about 700 ml of liquid effusion. Omental fatty tissue jelly-like. Thyroid normal size, yellowish grey, shiny in both lobes. One walnut size adenoma filled with colloid. Very small heart, 120 g, valves thin and smooth, aorta usual width, cardiac muscle well defined, reddish brown, solid, width 0.1 c in right atrium, 0.9 c in left atrium. Normal size lungs. When cut, fluffy greyish pink, lower lobes bloated. Increased number of tracheobronchial glands with small calcifications and chalky deposits. Small atrophic spleen, 70 g. Flat, normal size adrenals, cortex very narrow, brownish yellow. Medulla very narrow, greyish white. Small atrophic kidneys, 80 g each. Normal size liver with brown atrophy, 960 g. Gall bladder contains brown slightly syrupy gall and a few soft yellow brown disintegrating stones. Pancreas normal size, compact lobes visible, yellowish grey, 65 g. Sex organs normal. Stomach and intestines have smooth yellowish grey mucosa covered with a small amount of mucus. In the jejunum there are small petechiae. Bone marrow in right femur fatty.

Microscopic Study

Cerebrum: normal, in spots small glial proliferations in subependyma.

Cerebellum: normal, epiphysis normally built with a few calcifications.

Cardiac muscle: built normally, well marked striations. Next to nuclei very small groups of granules of brown pigment. In spots single nuclei bigger and darker stained.

Aorta: has thin wall, is built normally.

Lungs: alveolar build, well preserved, in places very thin walls. Some alveoli filled with fibers, neutrophil leukocytes, and big cells with round dark staining nuclei and sparse acidophilic plasma. In bronchi clusters of neutrophil leukocytes and mucus.

Spleen: capsule and trabeculae thick; hyaline changes. Lymph nodes sparse, sometimes very small, fibrous, and containing hyaline bodies in the center. Reticulum very profuse. In a few places small caseous trabecular spots. Granulations of small amounts of iron and blood pigment present mostly as very minute granules in reticular cells.

Skin: thin epidermis well differentiated from adjoining layers. Large amounts of melanin in basal and adjoining tissues. Thin granular and thicker keratin layer; papillary layer underdeveloped. In the dermis, mostly close to epidermis, small lymphocytic infiltrations of tunica adventitial origin around small capillaries. In spots several pigment carrying clumps of cells full of melanin.

Kidneys: glomeruli normal size. In spots many nuclei, in spots neutrophil single leukocytes, curved canaliculi, wide hexagonal epithelium slightly flattened, hyaline droplets associated with granulated or amorphous acidophils. Blood vessels are normal.

Liver: normally built with small vacuoles in principal cells. Intertrabecular crevices are narrow and contain only single RBCs or WBCs.

Pancreas: normally built. Islands of Langerhans composed of cells of different sizes and colors; some have very small nuclei, some have nuclei twice or three times normal size. Plasma cells are slightly granular or vacuolated. In spots in the region of the islets, there are empty amorphous spaces.

Adrenals: composed of foam cells in the glomeruli and in the exterior part of the band shaped layers. In the deeper layers are cells which stain with eosin and which contain small vacuoles. The medulla appear normal and contain islands of cortical tissue. In the cortex there is a single adenoma composed mostly of foam cells.

Parathyroids: normal. In spots there are clusters of cells with vacuoles filled with plasma. There are no alveolae.

Pituitary: normal. Basophil and eosinophil cells, singly or in small band shaped clusters, with prevalence of principal cells. Median lobe contains few adenomatous bodies. Posterior lobe normal.

Ovaries: contain some white bodies and numerous nonripe or ripening graffian follicles. In spots in the interstitium there are single large roundish cells, filled with brown pigment.

Lymphatic glands: generally normal with many typical small nodes, partially epithelial, with very small cheesy spots. In the glands of the mediastinum there are some bigger cheesy spots surrounded with tubercular granulations.

Nipple: has abundant interstitium, single diminutive glandular ducts, and no glandular acini at all.

Bone marrow: has fibrous connective tissue, numerous mostly band shaped cellular clusters with RBCs, some with nuclei. Myeloblasts and myelocytes and a few lymphocytes and leukocytes.

This is the case with extensive atrophy of the organs and emphysematic changes in lungs.

CASE 5

Male, age 39, autopsy 5½ hours after death. Clinical diagnosis: acute inanition. Anatomopathological diagnosis: fibrous superficial colitis, brown atrophy of the heart, acute inanition, gastritis, emphysema of the left lung. Synechia of the right lung.

From the Autopsy Report

Above normal height; very poor nutrition; build normal; hair light brown; skin thin, cadaverlike, pale, rather elastic, desquamating. Brain without macroscopic changes, weight 1480 g; ependyma of the lateral ventricle appears as though sprinkled with sand. Heart the size of the fist, 220 g. Contains some blood clots and liquid blood. Pericardium contains a little clear yellowish liquid below some gellike fat. Cavities usual width, valves thin and smooth. Cardiac muscle well differentiated, pinkish brown, usual consistency. Normal size lungs, rims connecting, normally collapsing, full of air when cut, greyish pink-black, slightly bloated. Mucopurulent liquid comes out of bronchi. Spleen usual size and shape, 230 g. Capsule slightly wrinkled when cut, dark pink interstitium clearly defined, no visible follicles, usual consistency. Adrenals normal size; flat; cortex narrow, yellowish brown; medulla narrow, grey. Right kidney 130 g, left 150 g, normal, slightly atrophic. Liver 1180 g, brown atrophy. Very small stomach, creased greyish pink mucosa, profusely covered with mucus. Sex organs macroscopically normal. Small intestines have some yellow brown liquid content. Mucosa smooth greyish pink. Large intestine contains a lot of feces, liquid and mushy. Mucosa greyish pink, lower parts covered with delicate fibers.

Microscopic Study

Brain: normal. In one spot aggregate of glia and single lymphocytes similar to typhus nodules. In a few places focal small glial proliferations containing single lymphocytes. In the walls of the cavities some papular excrescences covered with normal ependyma; in some places these excrescences contain proliferating glia. In some spots small aggregates of rod shaped cells around capillaries. Capillaries have edematous mesenthelium.

Epiphysis: normal, few calcifications.

Esophagus: built normally. In mucosa, under the epithelium, many clusters of lymphocytes, plasma cells with single neutrophils, and numerous blood filled capillaries.

Stomach: normal. Between glands numerous and profuse clusters of plasma cells, lymphocytes, and neutrophils. On the surface of the mucosa, a number of leukocytes and plasma cells, in between mucous mass. Desquamating surface layers of the epithelial layer of the mucosa.

Duodenum and small intestine: normally built. Infiltrations, desquamation, amassment of mucus as in the stomach. Small regular glandular ducts.

Large intestine: normally built. Many lymphocytes, plasma cells, and neutrophils between Lieberkuhn glands. Outlying layers of mucosa desquamating profusely. Surface covered with fibrous infiltrations, containing numerous leukocytes and plasma cells.

Cardiac muscle: normally built. Under pericardium some fatty atrophic tissue with occasional lipofuscin infiltrations. In the fibers dense nuclei sometimes with pyknotic changes and lipofuscin.

Lungs: filled with air. Very thin alveolar walls, in many spots coal deposits, large lumen. In alveoli some clusters of leukocytes.

Spleen: thick capsule built from fibrous conjunctive tissue. Medium size lymph nodes without proliferative foci. In the red pulp many RBCs, some with nuclei. Numerous thick trabeculae. Smaller vessels have extensive hyaline changes.

Skin: built normally. Very narrow and poorly developed epidermal papillary layer. Keratin layer broad. Poorly developed granular layer of the epidermis. In spots small infiltrations of lymphocytes and plasma cells in dermis, also clusters of cells containing pigment.

Kidneys: medium size normally built glomeruli; rather dense cells. In spots single leukocytes and lymphocytes. Capillaries very full. Some single glomeruli have hyaline changes. Epithelium of the curved canals is protruding slightly toward the lumen, with plasma containing a few hyaline droplets. Vessels have thick hyaline walls and very small lumen. The interstitium contains small lymphocytes, infiltrates, and colloidal sacks. The canaliculi, especially the curved ones, are prolapsed.

Liver: contains thin trabeculae with large lymphatic spaces and capillaries among them, with single WBCs and numerous RBCs. In the plasma randomly placed lipofuscins, mostly in the central part of the lobule. Some cells with two nuclei, some with big hyperchromic nuclei. In Kernan's cavities small clusters of lymphocytes and a thick capsule of fibrous conjunctive tissue.

Pancreas: built normally. Small alveolae and prolapsed ductus deferens. Numerous tiny islands of Langerhans. Plasma in cells almost invisible. Nuclei small, often pyknotic.

Left adrenal: has narrow cortex, three layers well differentiated. In the glomerular layer there are a small number of cells with foamy plasma; some of those also are present in the band shaped layer. Sparse brown pigment in the reticular layer, mostly close to the medulla. Medulla large and well preserved. In spots smaller and bigger islands and projections of the cortex. In spots, in the medulla and in the cortex in vicinity of medulla, small clusters of lymphocytes.

Right adrenal: similar to the left. In deeper layer of cortex in vicinity of medulla some cells filled with brown pigment are strewn in loose vascularized connective tissue. Lack of cells with fatty bodies. In one spot in cortex there are small adenomas built from this type of cell, but even they lack fatty bodies.

Thyroid: normal, medium size alveoli full of watery colloid slightly acidophilic with several round empty spaces. Besides thyroid lobes there are few somehow separated pieces with compact agglomerates of roundish or oval epithelial cells.

Parathyroids: normal. Plasma cells often do not take up stain. In spots smaller and larger cysts full of colloid.

Pituitary: normal build, cells mostly basophils and principals. Acidophils form tiny aggregates, mostly in peripheral parts of the pituitary, but some also in inner layers. Posterior part is normal. In spots small clusters of basophil and eosinophil cells. The central part is composed of a number of cysts lined with one layer of hexagonal or flat epithelium. In between cysts single or clustered cells from anterior part of the pituitary, mostly eosinophils.

Testes: the seminal canals are separated in many places by masses of loose connective tissue filled with cells. The seminal canals have very little sperm, but amorphous liquid slightly eosinophil. Spermatogenesis is limited; in some canals there is none. Very small mesenchymal cells, sometimes elongated with brown plasma, are visible only in spots. Mostly, they appear singly amidst loose connective tissue among canals. Epididymis is normal; its canals are prolapsed.

Lymphatic glands: have small nodes, devoid of signs of proliferation. In some spots sinusitis.

Striated muscles: generally normal, but thin fibers do not take the dye, and striations are hardly visible; in spots hyaline changes. Nuclei mostly pyknotic.

In this case atrophy is the most obvious of symptoms. Changes in brain are the same as those in typhus (petechial). Therefore we consider this case to be typhus without clinical symptoms, and obviously also hunger disease. The fresh and acute changes in intestines are probably pseudodysenteric. Bacteriological feces examination was negative. Lungs show emphysema.

CASE 6

Female 42 years old. Autopsy 38 hours after death. Clinical diagnosis: colitis, inanition, edema of the extremities. Anatomopathological diagnosis: fibrinous pseudomembranous dysentery, inanition, atrophy of organs, brown atrophy of liver and myocardium. Complete atrophy of fatty tissue. Emphysema. Red marrow bone of the right femur. Pleural adhesions, bilateral hydrothorax, ascites.

From the Autopsy Report

Height below normal, nutrition very poor, normal build, hair light brown. Skin brownish, thin, slightly desquamated, poorly elastic, a few lacunae on the abdomen. Cerebrum normal, 1240 g. Abdomen 2.5 liters, right pleural cavity 250 ml, left pleural cavity 1600 ml of fluid. Heart small, 160 g; jellylike fat under pericardium, heart cavities wider, valves smooth and thin. Cardiac muscle normally built, brownish, compact, right atrium wall 0.3 cm wide, left 1.0 cm. Regular size lungs, fluffy reddish grey when cut, scarified focus size of a hazelnut in the right apex. Small atrophic spleen, 70 g. Adrenals normal size, cortex narrow, yellowish grey, medulla narrow, grey-white. Small atrophic kidneys, right 110 g, left 120 g. Liver with brown atrophy, 800 g. Sex organs normal. Rather wide stomach contains yellowish grey liquid. Mucosa creased, greenish grey. Small intestines prolapsed, their mucosa covered with mucus, pale yellowish grey. In large intestines, in caecum, ascending colon, and transverse colon slightly edematous mucosa with tiny petechiae. Descending colon, sigmoid, and rectum have thick hard walls, thick mucosa, reddish, covered with fibrous membranes increasing toward the lower end. Bone marrow in right femur is sparse and red.

Microscopic Study

Brain: normal architecture; in some places around small vessels focal clusters of roundish cells with alveolar or darkly stained nuclei and very sparse eosinophilia. Often invisible cytoplasm. In lymphatic spaces around vessels clusters of lymphatic cells or sparse pigmentary yellow-gold infiltrations. No changes in cerebellum.

Large intestines: lack of regular mucosa. Instead of fibrous-necrotic effusion, masses and granulations with large number of leukocytes, neutrophils, lymphocytes, plasmatic cells, and large cells with roundish darkly staining nuclei and amorphous rather rich acidophil plasma, sometimes with vacuoles. In spots, amidst the granulations, remnants of intestinal glands, also amorphous mounds of chromatin in submucosa. Some infiltrates of lymphocytes, macrophages, and plasma cells. Muscular layer normal, few infiltrations. In mucous layer quite large clusters of infiltrations, similar to interstice.

Cardiac muscle: built normally. Fibers are narrow, striations well determined; around nuclei, spindlelike aggregates of finely granulated brownish pigment. In spots bigger aggregates of conjunctive tissue around vessels, sometimes with a few lymphocytes. In many places bigger, often shapeless hyperchromic nuclei. In certain parts the nuclei are dense, often with pyknotic changes.

Aorta: normal.

Lungs: generally normal. Vessels, including capillaries, are full of blood. Empty alveoli with very thin walls. In spots coal infiltration. Lack of iron pigment.

Spleen: very thick trabecule and capsule with hyaline changes. Lymph nodes quite numerous, very small, without proliferation center. Their vessels have very thin lumen, thick hyaline walls. In the red pulp large infiltrations of hemosiderin contained in granules of varying size in the sinus walls, and also in loose cells lying in sinuses.

Skin: very thin epidermis, not very well separated from interstice. In basal cell layer a lot of melanin. Keratin layer broad. Almost no granulated layer only keratohyaline granules in spots. Slightly developed papillary layer. Under epidermis very many pigment carrying cells full of melanin. In dermis around capillaries many small clusters of cells of tunica adventitial origin or of lymphocytes.

Kidneys: generally normal, small glomerulae. In Bowman's capsules serous liquid. In epithelium of curved canals hyaline droplets. Canals are wide with flat epithelia, full of eosinophils or vacuoles. Vessels have normal structure with hyaline changes in spots. Kidneys are very well supplied with blood.

Liver: normal except for small lobule and thin trabeculae. In broad intratrabecular spaces numerous RBCs and lymphocytes. Liver cells are small, often with very tiny darkly stained nuclei. In many cells the nuclei are twice as big and hyperchromic. In the plasma of the cells in the central part as well as on the periphery of the lobule there are granules of lipofuscin. In the interlobular spaces some vessels have thick walls with hyaline changes and in some places there are small clusters of lymphocytes.

Pancreas: built normally. In the head few islands of Langerhans composed of roundish cells with small, round, uniformly stained dark nuclei and in spots with vacuole plasma. In some places within islands there are large empty shapeless spaces, so that the island looks like a tube. In the tail part of the pancreas there are more islands, bigger than those in the head part.

Adrenals: right is long, flat, its structure well preserved. In the cortex the strongest is band shaped layer. Its cells as well as cells in glomerular layer are mostly foamy. Medulla is normally well developed. It contains some cortex originated islands and in spots medium clumps of lymphocytes. Left adrenal has very poorly developed medulla, and in the cortex many cells have acidophil plasma, almost devoid of foamy aspect.

Parathyroids: small, normal, devoid of colloidal alveoli, and have good blood supply.

Pituitary: has very good blood supply. Eosinophil cells form smaller and bigger aggregates. Basophil cells are rather plentiful in very small clusters. Principal cells prevalent. In central part few cysts filled with slightly acidophil and granulated content. In the posterior part profuse infiltrations of brown pigment.

Ovaries: have very many whitish bodies. Their vessels have very thick walls, small lumen, pronounced hyalinic changes. In some places in mesenchymal tissue there are big, single, shapeless cells filled with brown or gold melaninlike pigment.

Nipple: among solid hyalinelike conjunctive tissue there are some small sparse parts of tubes and glands, rarely clumped into bigger groups. In spots there are adenomatous bodies lined with low basophil epithelium as well as tall eosinophil epithelium like sweat glands.

Bone marrow: is composed of fibrous conjunctive tissue sparsely strewn with small clusters of RBCs, partially containing nuclei and myelocystic and myeloblastic cells. Very few lymphocytes and leukocytes.

Striated muscles: have very thin fibers not uniformly stained. Striations are hardly visible in some places. In many places number of nuclei is increased; in some places few nuclei are clustered together. In spots there are shapeless darkly stained chromatin masses; in spots muscular fibers are hyalinized or granularly necrotic.

In this case we have advanced atrophic changes. Symptoms in the large intestine are identical to dysenteric symptoms, but bacteriological examination of feces was negative. Large amount of hemosiderin in spleen. Lungs emphysemic.

INDEX

Absorption, 72, 101
Acid base balance, 88-94, 119
  chloride metabolism, 88-89, 115
Acidosis, 121-122
  diabetic, 73
Addison's disease, 106-107, 165, 234
Adrenalin, 21, 31, 55, 65, 71, 73, 76, 79-81,
  84, 93, 112
Adrenals, 76, 106-107, 111-112, 200, 210,
  221-222, 225-226, 233-234
Albumin, 42, 71, 106-107
Alcohol load, 90
Aldrich-McClure water test, 17-18, 39, 49,
  60, 97, 121-122
Allergic diseases, 22
  asthma, 22, 40, 56, 65
  enteritis, 22
  food allergy, 22, 40
  gastritis, 22
  hay fever, 22, 40
  rheumatic fever, 65
  serum sickness, 56, 65
  urticaria, 22, 40
Amino acids, 95
  cysteine, 22, 95
  cystine, 22, 95
  glutathione, 95
Amyloidosis, 22, 229
Anemia, 30, 41, 53, 63, 159, 165, 167, 173,
  190, 215, 233
  hyperchromic, 163, 166, 185
  hypochromic, 30, 163, 166, 185
  normochromic, 166

pernicious, 163, 167, 192
Aneurin, 73
Angulus infectiosus oris, 19, 104
Anti-insulin factors, 79, 83-84, 117
Archard cavities, 22
Atherosclerosis, 41
Autonomic nervous system, 23, 25, 55, 65,
  112-114, 159-160
  adrenergic system, 26, 55, 112-113, 152,
  159
  cholinergic system, 26, 55, 112-114, 152,
  159
  hypoamphotony, 26
  ocular pressure test, 25, 113
  pharmacological stimulation, 25
    with adrenalin, 25
    with atropine, 25
    with pilocarpin, 25, 113
  salivation, 25, 55
  sweating, 25, 55
  tremor, 25
  vagus nerve, 32, 55, 65
Autopsy case reports, 237-254

Bang, 75
Banting, 74
Basal metabolism, 84-88, 105-107, 110,
  117, 121, 123, 127, 132, 134-135,
  138, 147, 149-152, 154, 157, 159-
  160
Benedict, 74, 85
Best, 74
Beta lipoproteins, 42